How to Heal
Yeast Infections
Naturally

A Holistic Approach to
Curing Candida Overgrowth

Murielle L. DuBois, ND,RHN

May this book help you find peace,

healing, and renewed

vitality

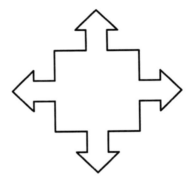

Acknowledgements

This book is lovingly dedicated
to the memory of my father, Simon DuBois, who
once said to me when I was a child,
"Murielle, take care of your health!"

Also, I wish to acknowledge and thank those people who have been my teachers and mentors and who have helped me to continually refine my natural health mindset. Thank you to Jane Beresford, my mother, who taught me by example, for her patience and encouragement.

Thank you to Randy Peyser at www.AuthorOneStop.com for her guidance in writing this book.

This book is dedicated to the women who knowingly or unknowingly suffer from the minor or major mental, emotional, and physical discomforts of *Candida* yeast overgrowth. May my book help you find peace, healing, and renewed vitality!

Table of Contents

Preface

Health is my passion, and I want to share with you my knowledge and personal experience with yeast infections. I finally found a solution to keep them under control, and I want to share it with the whole world! I want women to know that they don't have to suffer with yeast infections, and they don't need to use Canesten (the brand name for Clotrimazole, a common antifungal medication). There are healthier alternatives!

As a result of reading this book, you will:

- Learn how to cure your yeast infection with a holistic approach

- Learn what to do about *Candida albicans*

- Learn how to get off of "pain island"

- Learn specific ideas about what works best for you

- Stop suffering from yeast infections

- Eliminate Canesten and take control over your health

- Overcome objections to "I don't know how"

- Discover the answers to common questions about yeast infections

- Learn what the makers of Canesten might not tell you

- Learn what a yeast infection is and its possible causes

- Recognize symptoms of a yeast infection and eliminate them in twelve hours

- Learn if it is safe to have sex while suffering from a yeast infection

- Learn about food sensitivities and alternatives

- Stay healthy despite stress, and regain your lost energy and vitality

- Be in harmony with your mind, body, and soul

- Improve your health and pursue activities you enjoy

The doctor of the future will give no medicine but

will interest his patients in the care of the human frame,

in proper diet, and in the cause and prevention of disease.

—Thomas A. Edison

Chapter 1

Candida

There are many yeast infections books on the market. While some offer valuable guidance, others offer confusing and contradictory information. I find that my experience and research stand alone as the most updated, comprehensive, and down-to-earth book on *Candida*, and I personally can testify that my recommendations work. This book provides in-depth research into the underlying causes of *Candida* overgrowth, and covers prevention, treatment, and diet. I have followed these diet recommendations and taken some antifungal treatments and brought my *Candida* level from 7 to 2.

Are you ready to learn about *Candida* so you won't need to use Canesten and other drugs anymore? On the following pages, you will learn the best ways to cure your yeast infection naturally.

What Is Yeast?

Yeasts are simple (single-celled) organisms belonging to the vegetable kingdom. They are extremely common in our environment, living in soil and on fruits and vegetables, thriving wherever there is decay, and floating in the air we breathe. Mold is a type of yeast.

One type of yeast that lives in our bodies is called *Candida albicans* (*C. albicans*). All of us carry *Candida* at all times, especially in the digestive tract and the vagina, and most of the time it exists in harmony with the multitude of other bacteria and microbes we carry. Sometimes, though, *Candida* proliferates and disrupts the normal balance of microbes, setting the stage for a variety of health problems.

There are three types of vaginal infections, or vaginitis. Trichomoniasis is a vaginal infection triggered by parasitic protozoa; bacterial vaginosis is a vaginal infection often transmitted sexually and caused by bacteria; and a yeast infection, known as candidiasis, is a vaginal infection caused by yeast-like microorganisms such as *C. albicans*.

Factors that Contribute to the Overgrowth of *Candida*

An important factor in controlling the levels of *Candida* in the body is the presence of several types of bacteria, including *Lactobacillus acidophilus*. This bacteria takes the main food of *Candida*, glucose, and turns it into lactic acid, thus inhibiting overgrowth of the yeast. If you take antibiotics then you are likely to kill off the bacteria in your body, good and bad. This permits *Candida* to grow unchecked, and if you take repeat prescriptions of antibiotics you can rapidly enter a state of *Candida* proliferation and experience health problems relating to it.

Candida colonizes the mucus membranes that line the digestive tract and vagina. These membranes produce a thick mucus that is both protective and lubricating. If the glucose content of the mucus is allowed to rise, then the *Candida* flourishes. The major way that this comes about is through taking in too many refined carbohydrates (white-flour products, candies, and soft drinks). These are very rapidly absorbed from the gut and find their way to the mucus to form food for the yeast. Other sugary foods that may aggravate the problem include fruits and alcohol.

Fluctuations in hormonal levels can affect the growth of *Candida*. Thus, during pregnancy and with the use of the contraceptive pill, a woman is more likely to suffer from *Candida* overgrowth. At certain times during the menstrual cycle (in the week or so just prior to menstruation), as a woman's pH changes, the hormonal picture is also favorable to *Candida*. Women are more susceptible to these infections than men because a woman's monthly hormone cycle alters the body's pH, providing a better environment for yeast to thrive.

The use of douches as a means of personal hygiene may aggravate vaginal growth of *Candida* because the beneficial *Lactobacillus* is washed away. Women should especially avoid scented or perfumed products because they may be irritating.

An impaired immune system will predispose a woman to *Candida* colonization, which can occur due to a number of other factors:

- Prolonged or extreme stress
- Nutritional deficiencies
- Allergies to foods or environmental factors
- Prolonged use of prescription drugs
- Chronic illnesses
- Prolonged fatigue
- Use of alcohol and recreational drugs
- A high-sugar and -starch diet

What Is *Candida*?

Many people think that yeast infections only occur in females and are primarily a vaginal infection. But *Candida* also affects men and children alike. Its main habitat is the digestive tract. Fungi are everywhere and exist in a balanced state in the human body until we disrupt the balance through the use of antibiotics or cortisone, or by excess sugar consumption.

Small amounts of yeast and other fungal organisms compose a normal part of the body's microflora. They normally are well tolerated by those with healthy immunity. If they increase in number, however, they create additional stress to the immune system, which can lead to an overgrowth. Those with weakened immune systems become susceptible to overgrowth of *C. albicans*. The growth of yeasts is normally kept in check in the intestinal system by the presence of *L. acidophilus* and other beneficial bacteria.

Women most susceptible to *Candida* overgrowth are those with allergies, poor digestion, and other diseases or illnesses; histories of long treatments of antibiotics, birth-control pills, or other drugs; or those who are under excessive stress, are overtired, or overworked. *Candida* overgrowth can be found in women who are doers, givers, overachievers, workaholics, have low self-esteem, or who spread themselves too thin.

An overabundance of yeast in the body can produce side effects including anxiety, allergies, asthma, acne, bloating, cystitis, chemical sensitivities, coughs, cramps, constipation, chronic fatigue syndrome, confusion, trouble concentrating, depression, diarrhea, emotional problems, eczema, fatigue, fuzzy thinking, food cravings and sensitivities, gas, indigestion, headaches, hypoglycemia, hives, hyperactivity, heartburn, irritability, indigestion, intestinal pain, irrational fears, lethargy, low self-esteem, memory loss or poor memory, migraines, sore muscles, nausea, panic, puffiness, PMS, psoriasis, quick anger, rash, skin infections, stiffness, sleep disturbance, sinus pressure, sore throat, thrush, vaginal yeast infections, and weight gain.

When we disrupt the normal flora balance with antibiotics (penicillin, tetracycline, erythromycin, sulfa drugs, and many others), immunosuppressive drugs such as chemotherapy, or steroid drugs such as estrogens, the birth-control pill, progesterone, or cortisone, we create an imbalance in the bowel which favors the growth of fungi. Stress, diabetes, hypoglycaemia, and other metabolic diseases can be triggers for *Candida* or another fungal proliferation, leading to infection, inflammation, and chronic disease.

Consuming large amounts of refined carbohydrates (candies, chocolate, cakes, cookies, chips, soft drinks, white breads, donuts), alcohol, and caffeine leads to excessive growth of fungi. Even the sugar found in fruits and fruit juices, if consumed in large enough amounts, can favor the overgrowth of gastrointestinal fungi. Yeast and fungi thrive in the gastrointestinal tract when provided with large doses of sugar in almost any form.

Diabetics frequently suffer from the effects of an overgrowth of yeast, particularly when blood-sugar levels are not under control. Many diseases in which the immune system is compromised are associated with yeast infections. *Candida* seems to thrive whenever the immune system has been weakened by drugs, disease, or poor diet. The mercury found in the common black dental filling has been implicated as an immunosuppressive agent. A large number of scientific studies link fungal infections with silver mercury dental amalgam hypersensitivity. Stress, chemical additives, and nutritional deficiencies create an overgrowth of yeast in the colon. The yeast spreads up in the digestive tract into the small intestine, stomach, esophagus, and oral cavity. In the mouth, *Candida* infection produces a noticeable white coating of the mucus membranes known as thrush. The tongue, gums, cheeks, and palate may all be coated with *Candida* or other fungi.

Mycotoxins: Source of the Symptoms

Candida and other fungi produce a large number of biologically active substances called mycotoxins. These toxins are secreted to serve the fungus by protecting it against viruses, bacteria, parasites like protozoa, insects, animals, and humans. In the human host, these toxins can get into the bloodstream and produce an array of central nervous system symptoms (fatigue, confusion, irritability, mental fogginess, memory loss, depression, dizziness, mood swings, headaches, nausea, burning sensations, numbness, tingling, and others).

Fungal problems are usually secondary to other primary imbalances related to the general health of the immune and endocrine system. Treating only the fungal infection may help relieve symptoms, but it may not necessarily relieve the primary defect (for example, diabetes, adrenal insufficiency, vitamin and mineral deficiencies, immune dysfunction, toxic heavy metal poisoning—especially with mercury—hydrochloric acid deficiency, pancreatic enzyme deficiency, hypothyroidism, and others). Ideally, this could be sorted out by tests ordered by a healthcare practitioner.

A lack of hydrochloric acid production by the stomach (a condition called achlorhydria) or an insufficiency of this acid (hydrochlorhydria) predisposes an individual to *Candida* or fungal overgrowth. In healthy individuals, the high acid content of gastric juices helps kill off most fungi and other potentially harmful microorganisms found in food. As one grows older and the stomach's ability to produce hydrochloric acid diminishes, however, *Candida* and other fungi can get past the stomach acid barrier and overpopulate the gut. One of the major inhibitors of hydrochloric acid production is an unsuspected food allergy, especially to wheat or dairy products. The problem can be reversed by eliminating the offending allergic foods and improving the diet with acidifying nutritional supplements.

Pancreatic enzyme deficiency can cause fungal overgrowth in the gastrointestinal tract. Like hydrochloric acid, pancreatic enzymes (protease, lipase, amylase, and others) help digest and inactivate fungi that enter the body with food. Low stomach acid production and pancreatic enzyme insufficiency can be diagnosed through a comprehensive stool and digestive analysis ordered by a natural healthcare practitioner. Acid or pancreatic digestive enzyme supplements can be taken to improve the situation. Examples of acid and other digestive enzyme supplements include glutamic acid, betaine hydrochloride, pepsin, pancreatin, bile salts, papain, bromelain, stomach bitters, and plant enzymes.

Evidence now exists that fungi, through production of mycotoxins, initiate many degenerative diseases: cancer, heart disease, gout, arthritis, and autoimmune disease (thyroiditis, chronic fatigue syndrome, multiple sclerosis, systemic lupus erythematosus, rheumatoid arthritis, myasthenia gravis, scleroderma, and others). The major fatal diseases in North America are intimately connected to fungal mycotoxins.

Many foods typically considered healthful have been discovered to be heavily colonized by fungi and their mycotoxins. These include corn, peanuts, cashews, and dried coconut. To a lesser degree, fungi can also be found in breads of all kinds, in flours made from barley, rye, wheat, rice, millet, and practically all cereal grains. A diet high in contaminated grains and nuts increases the likelihood of fungal colonization of the gastrointestinal tract. Worse, animals fed mycotoxin-contaminated grains end up with fungal overgrowth; the fat and muscles of most grain-fed animals in North America are loaded with mycotoxins.

Animal fat has been well documented to be associated with a greater risk of both heart disease and cancer. According to some researchers, it is not the animal fat that increases cancer and heart-disease risk, it is the mycotoxin load in the fat itself.

We have all been brought up with the unshakable dogma that cigarette smoking causes lung cancer and that tobacco is a carcinogen. Few realize that all the cigarettes sold in North America are contaminated with yeast or fungi and have had sugar and yeast added to the final product. Sugar increases fungal growth. So does baker's or brewer's yeast. It is conceivable that tobacco itself is harmless and that it is made carcinogenic commercially, partially because of the fungal contamination. The mycotoxin fusarium, found in cigarettes, has been linked with lung cancer, esophageal cancer, and cancer of the uterus. The manufacture of bread, beer, wine, cheese, chewing tobacco, aged and cured meats, and cigarettes involves a fungal fermentation process and increases the likelihood of exposure to mycotoxins. Alcohol is a fungal-produced toxin, and has been documented to cause brain and nervous system damage, liver cancer, birth defects, and hundreds of other negative health conditions. The consumption of small amounts of these foods may be tolerated by those with healthy immune systems but deadly to those suffering from chronic illness of any kind.

Western diets contain factors that encourage the growth of yeast. Antibiotics are used in animal feed, especially for poultry, pork, and beef intended for human consumption. Trace amounts of these antibiotics are found in most of the meats we eat, meaning that each of us is exposed to these drugs every day, even when we're not taking them for an infection. Antibiotics are "blind bullets" that can't tell the harmful bacteria from the healthy ones. Instead of just killing microorganisms that cause infection, they also kill the *Lactobacillus acidophilus* that grows in the gut. These colon bacteria form a first line of defense for us, producing acid that keeps both yeast and certain harmful bacteria from living inside us. When the "good" bugs are killed, yeast can begin to grow out of balance on the inside, in the gut. When the yeast toxin damages the defense system, the body cannot kill the new invaders.

So it's not just the antibiotics we take; it is also those given to the animals we eventually eat. Animals are given antibiotics to treat and prevent infection, but there's more: Some antibiotics stimulate growth in animals. Ranchers and producers who want to fatten their profits may use antibiotics to fatten their animals. If you eat a lot of meat that contains even traces of antibiotics, you may develop a bacteria–yeast imbalance in your intestines.

Candida produces several toxic waste substances. When acetaldehyde, the main toxic waste of *Candida*, transforms into ethanol, it can cause a variety of unpleasant symptoms, including oral thrush, vaginal yeast infection, upper back pain, bloating, diarrhea, constipation, GERD, heartburn, sores in the anus, brain fog, dental problems, TMJ, migraines, blurred vision, depression, restless leg syndrome, panic attacks, chronic athlete's foot, high cholesterol, and asthma.

Chapter 2
The Symptoms of Candida Overgrowth

Candida normally exists in the body in the form of spores. These cannot cross the barrier of the mucus membrane and thus cause only local symptoms when they proliferate. But if *Candida* growth is unchecked, eventually the spores develop into the mycelial form, which means that instead of being individual single cells, they begin to clump together and form long strands. These can penetrate the intestinal and vaginal walls and can enter the bloodstream to be disseminated throughout the body.

Initially, symptoms of *Candida* overgrowth are confined to the digestive system (usually the lower bowel), the vagina in women, and the urethra and prostate gland in men. But later, as the yeast proliferates and spreads through the body, the symptoms can affect many different parts of the body.

Primary factors that lead to *Candida* overgrowth include:

- Poor dietary choices and compromised digestion
- Weakened immune system
- Improper acid-alkaline balance or imbalance of digestive enzymes
- Accumulation of toxins in the digestive tract
- The loss of friendly probiotic bacteria

The first and most obvious sign that you may be getting a vaginal yeast infection is discomfort in your vaginal area. You might feel itching or soreness around your labia and the entrance of your vagina. You might also feel a little swollen or redness. Other common symptoms (in no particular order) include:

- Recurrent vaginal infections (itching and whitish discharge that looks a little bit like cottage cheese)
- Burning sensation when you urinate, and pain or burning sensation during sexual intercourse
- Menstrual disruption (especially PMS)
- Cyclic vulvovaginitis: recurrent pain, burning and itching sensation during every menstrual cycle
- Fatigue or chronic fatigue, especially after eating
- Depression
- Irritability
- Sensitivity to tobacco smoke, cigarettes
- Abdominal pain and distention
- Rectal itching
- Recurrent vaginal or urinary infections
- Prostatis
- Symptoms that are worse on damp, muggy days or in moldy places (basements or damp climates)
- Adverse neurological effects of "sick building syndrome" caused by mold in the environment
- Heartburn and indigestion

- Muscle and joint pain
- Tingling and weakness of the limbs
- Blurred vision or spots in front of the eyes ("floaters" in the eyes)
- Hypoglycaemia
- Headaches
- "Spacing out" (brain fog)
- Loss of memory and/or concentration
- Arthritis
- Impotence or reduced sex drive
- Sinus problems
- Urinary disorders
- Frequent urination
- Hyperactivity
- Cold hands or feet and /or chilliness
- Learning difficulties
- Nasal congestion, sinusitis, or sinus infection
- Respiratory disorders
- Fungal infections of the nails
- Constipation or diarrhea
- Skin rashes, acne, rosacea, eczema, psoriasis

Esophageal candidiasis can cause difficulty swallowing, heartburn, the feeling of pain behind the breastbone, and nausea or vomiting.

Yeast infection symptoms vary and often change as the infection develops. Each of us has different *Candida* infection severities, different levels of immune system strength, different levels of healthy probiotics, varying levels of stress, and other individual factors that affect the ability of *Candida* to multiply and to cause harm.

Sometimes you have to try more than one treatment to find out what works best for you. Each person is unique in adapting and reacting to the treatments. There is no quick fix. A long-term solution to *Candida* overgrowth requires several steps and lifestyle changes.

Yeast infection is triggered by more than one factor, which makes it difficult to get under control. This one of the reasons why doctors might find *Candida* hard to eliminate using prescription and over-the-counter drugs. The holistic way might tackle the problem at the root and restore the inner environment back into balance.

Stress

Stress produced by lack of sleep, emotional issues, anxiety, or pressure in your daily routine has been proven to trigger yeast infection growth due to the following reasons:

➤ Stress depresses your immune system, since at the time of stress your body releases a hormone called cortisol, making your body defenseless against *Candida*.
➤ Stress elevates blood sugar levels that feed *Candida* cells, allowing them to overgrow.
➤ Stress changes our internal bacterial environment in the gut as it decreases the friendly bacteria, allowing overgrowth of *Candida*.

Hormonal Imbalance

Hormonal swings triggered by conditions like puberty, pregnancy, menstruation, PMS, and the use of oral contraceptives create a favorable environment for candidiasis. This is one of the reasons why many women often experience vaginal yeast infection during pregnancy and menstruation. During this time, the body goes through many hormonal fluctuations and changes in the vaginal acidity (pH levels), both of which could contribute to *Candida* overgrowth.

Chapter 3
Candida albicans and Allergies

Candida sets the stage for allergies.

A *Candida* overgrowth might cause and aggravate allergies in two ways:

1. Injecting the system with allergens that the *Candida* itself might produce.
2. Possibly causing a leaky gut. Yeast allergens produce classical allergic responses, causing symptoms such as itching, hives, skin rashes, nasal congestion, cough, bronchitis, irritable bowel, and asthma.

History and Symptoms of Fungal-Related Complex

- History of frequent antibiotics (healthy bacterial colonies in the intestines can usually withstand one or two short episodes of antibiotics without serious harm, depending on the individual)

- Persistent vaginitis, cystitis, or prostate or other genitor-urinary infections
- History of using birth-control pills, female hormone-replacement therapy, or cortisone-like drugs (cortisone or corticosteroids prescribed for skin conditions such as rashes, eczema, or psoriasis, or for systemic conditions such as rheumatoid arthritis)
- Reactions to perfumes, tobacco, insecticides, fabric shop odors, and other chemicals
- Development of multiple food and chemical allergies
- Athlete's foot, ringworm, jock itch, and chronic fungal, nail, or skin infections
- Chronic rashes or itching, psoriasis, or alcoholic beverages
- Fatigue, spaciness, lethargy, poor memory, numbness, tingling, burning
- Insomnia, muscle aches, weakness, paralysis, or joint pain or swelling
- Dry mouth or throat, rash or blisters in the mouth, bad breath
- Nasal congestion or post-nasal drip, nasal itching, sore throat, recurrent cough
- Bronchitis, laryngitis, wheezing, ear infections (otitis) or ear pain (otalgia)
- Immune-damaging illnesses such as diabetes
- Suppressed immune system from HIV/AIDS, chemotherapy, or organ transplant
- Abdominal pain, bloating, gas, diarrhea, constipation, and poor digestion
- Rectal itching, heartburn, food hypersensitivity, mucus in the stools
- Impotence, loss of libido, endometriosis, infertility, premenstrual syndrome
- Anxiety, depression, irritability, cold extremities, drowsiness, incoordination, mood swings
- Joint problems

- Irritable bowel syndrome
- Headaches, dizziness, tightness in chest, shortness of breath
- Foot, hair, or body odor not relieved by washing
- Fingernail and toenail infections
- Diaper rash and thrush in infants

Candida overgrowth can be triggered at a very young age when children are first being treated with antibiotics.

Genital Yeast Infection

Localized vaginal yeast infection symptoms include:

- ❖ Itching, irritation, and burning of the vagina or vulva
- ❖ White and abnormal discharge from the vagina
- ❖ Pain during sexual intercourse
- ❖ Inflammatory redness in the perineum area
- ❖ Oversensitivity and irritation of the pubic hair follicles
- ❖ Frequent pain during urination
- ❖ Low pelvic aching

Systemic vaginal yeast infection symptoms include:

- ❖ Severe swelling of the vagina characterized by a swollen anus and purple color of the vulva
- ❖ Pain during urination
- ❖ Painful skin cracks due to extreme dryness of the vaginal and vulva areas
- ❖ General fatigue and lethargy
- ❖ Walking difficulties
- ❖ Bloody exudation caused by scratching the area

❖ Bleeding and swelling of hemorroid veins
❖ Difficulties having sexual intercourse

Systemic *Candida* problems include: fever, heart murmur, enlargement of the spleen, bleeding disorders, infection in the eye area, and kidney problems.

There are some normal discharges during the menstrual cycle that are yellowish and mucus-like in consistency, and there are normal discharges when sexual arousal occurs. It's only when you seem to have white, cottage-cheese-like discharge, often accompanied by a bready or yeasty odor and several of the symptoms above, that you may suspect a yeast infection.

The fungal-related complex manifests primarily in five areas of the body:

1. **Digestive System**
   Symptoms include bloating, gas, cramps, alternating diarrhea with constipation, or multiple food allergies.

2. **Nervous System**
   Symptoms include abnormal fatigue, spaciness, anxiety, mood swings, drowsiness, memory loss, depression, insomnia, and/or mental fogginess. In extreme cases, hallucinations and violent behavior can occur. Autism, hyperactivity, and learning disabilities in children can be manifestations of fungal infestation.

3. **Skin**
   Symptoms include hives, psoriasis, eczema, excessive sweating, acne, and nail infections.

4. **Genito-Urinary Tract**
   In women, common problems include premenstrual syndrome (depression, mood swings, bloating, fluid retention, cramps,

craving for sweets, and headaches prior to menstruation), recurrent bladder or vaginal infections, and a loss of interest in sex. In males, common problems include chronic rectal or anal itching, recurrent prostatitis, impotence, genital rashes, and jock itch.

5. **Endocrine System**

Intimate relationships exist among the body's immune, nervous, and endocrine systems. The thyroid and adrenal glands in particular may be involved. Both hypo- and hyperthyroidism, especially the autoimmune variety, are strongly linked to fungal overgrowth.

Boosting Thymus Gland Function

The thymus gland is the largest gland of the immune system. There might be a direct link between *Candida* infection and compromised thymus gland function. The thymus gland is responsible of the production of T lymphocytes (T cells), the white blood cell responsible for cell-mediated immunity—the immune system function that protects against *C. albicans*, other fungi, viruses, and bacteria. The thymus gland is also responsible for the release of several hormones that regulate numerous immune functions. These hormone levels are usually low among individuals who suffer from infections, AIDS, and cancer.

Deficiencies in B vitamins, zinc, and vitamin C can result in a compromised production of immune beneficial hormones.

Candida and fungal toxins can travel to virtually all organs and tissues in the body. The syndrome has been associated with practically every medical condition, including cancer, heart disease, multiple sclerosis, AIDS, asthma, arthritis, chronic sinusitis, recurrent flu, middle ear infection, alcoholism, addiction, diabetes, eating disorders, hypoglycemia, and many other less-common conditions. A healthy immune system is the only natural defense against these microbes and their poisons.

A person's overall health must be enhanced by better nutrition, reduced stress, cigarette and alcohol cessation, exercise, spiritual and psychological therapy, and a less contaminated, less polluted environment. Dietary changes alone do not reverse *Candida* or fungal syndromes. Aggressive antifungal therapy might be necessary in some cases.

Chapter 4

Do You Have Candida albicans?

The most troublesome aspect of this syndrome is the diagnosis. Often, medical doctors are skeptical of *Candida* or the fungal complex and frequently point out that there are no unequivocally objective tests to verify its existence. Few doctors actively treat fungal and yeast infections, other than simple cases like jock itch, athlete's foot, and nail infections.

However, naturopathic doctors (NDs) can help you. They use tests to help diagnose *Candida* or fungal infections. Some of these have included the use of symptom questionnaires, skin tests, RAST or ELISA blood tests, and stool analysis.

Nonmedical practitioners may use electro-acupuncture techniques like Vega testing to diagnose *Candida*. Others use iridology, muscle testing, pendulum swinging, and radionics.

Candida questionnaires of all kinds might overdiagnose the problem. Lab tests (scratch test, serum RAST, serum antibody complexes, stool analysis, and others) used to detect the presence of *Candida* or fungi are associated with many false positives and negatives. *Candida* is normally an inhabitant of the gastrointestinal tract and skin of even the healthiest individuals, so a positive result on a lab test might not be definitive. As for the long list of nonmedical *Candida* tests, correlation with treatment outcomes has not been documented.

Some lab tests can indirectly show the presence of fungi in our bodies. Uric acid is not manufactured by the human body, despite what some medical texts claim and what most doctors believe. Fungi, on the other hand, have been proven able to manufacture uric acid. If blood tests show elevated uric acid in the body, this is nearly always a sign of fungal overgrowth or infections in the body. The use of antifungal therapy lowers the uric acid blood levels, further supporting the theory that high uric acid blood levels and gout are really the end result of fungal invasion. A normal or low uric acid blood level, however, is no guarantee of a negative diagnosis (that is, no infection).

There is no universal agreement about the relative merits of any single *Candida* or fungal test, save direct microscopic examination of blood or biopsied tissue. Live-cell microscopy is a test that offers a quick, reliable means of visualizing *Candida*, parasites, bacteria, other organisms, and their debris in live whole blood. One drop of blood from a fingertip puncture clearly shows living organisms floating freely in the bloodstream when examined with a microscope attached to a high-quality color video camera connected to a color monitor and video recorder. Live-cell microscopy, pioneered by Canadian scientist Gaston Naessens, creator of the 714X alternative cancer treatment, can reveal some health and disease data not possible through conventional microscopy.

The symptom that consistently appears in an otherwise medically healthy individual as a reliable indicator for trial therapy of antifungals is debilitating fatigue accompanied by spaciness or short-term memory loss.

The cholesterol in our blood does not come from dietary sources. Eating cholesterol does not cause heart disease. Cholesterol is a fat made by the body in response to the presence of fungal mycotoxins. It is a sign that something is wrong, not that it has to be lowered by reducing the cholesterol intake in the diet. The more fungal mycotoxins in the body, the more the liver will manufacture cholesterol to help neutralize the toxins. Studies indicate that following a high-sugar and -yeast diet (eating lots of bread and desserts) increases the *Candida* or fungal population in the gastrointestinal tract, elevates cholesterol, and increases the risk of heart disease.

The real role of the cholesterol in the body is to serve as a defense against mycotoxins. Cholesterol reduces the toxicity of mycotoxins by helping bind (chelate) them. In other words, high blood fats (hyperlipidemia) are protective. For this reason, a high blood level of cholesterol is a sign of fungal overgrowth or infection. Studies support the fact that use of antifungal therapies lowers cholesterol and reverses atherosclerosis. A normal cholesterol level does not necessarily indicate any fungal infection. A cholesterol level well below the normal reference range (below 150) might also be connected to fungal infections. In view of the confusion in both the medical and lay literature, the cholesterol–fungal connection is a concept that may take many years to accept.

If you suffer from one of the many autoimmune diseases like lupus, rheumatoid arthritis, thyroiditis, multiple sclerosis, colitis, or Crohn's disease, your treatment may be incomplete without attention to hidden fungal infections. In cases of chronic illness, especially in allergic conditions like hay fever, asthma, psoriasis, and eczema, candidal or fungal infestation may well be the culprit, causing the seemingly never-ending symptoms. A trial therapy with antifungal remedies might make all the difference to a complete recovery. Since the majority of these treatments are quite harmless, people with chronic immune system impairment can only win by complementing their medical or naturopathic treatments with an antifungal program.

Chronic Fungal or Vaginitis

Does your yeast infection keep coming back? Chronic fungal or candidal vaginitis does not always show up on cultures. In fact, cultures are a poor way of making the diagnosis. The problem is usually systemic and requires more than just the dietary approach of a yeast- and sugar-free diet and natural antifungals. Such cases sometimes require prescription antifungal medication. Ketoconazole (Nizoral) sometimes need to be used. Other options include fluconazole (Diflucan), itraconazole (Sporanox) and nystatin (Nilstat). If necessary, those drugs have to be taken.

Women with chronic fungal vaginitis should be assessed for hormonal imbalances, especially for a deficiency in progesterone and thyroid hormone. Calendula cream and vitamin E oil might be soothing for genital area irritation.

Food and chemical allergies are common in chronic inflammatory conditions.

Natural remedies applicable in chronic fungal vaginitis are: dong quai, Ginseng, black cohosh, flaxseed oil, evening primrose oil, borage oil, tea tree oil, *Lactobacillus acidophilus* and *bifidus*, boron, zinc, selenium, vitamin A, vitamin B6, and vitamin E.

A naturopath or holistic medical doctor can prescribe and supervise a personalized program.

Rate Your Health

Adults and teenagers can take this simple one-minute quiz for the yeast syndrome. Answer yes or no to the following questions. If you have four or five yes answers, you may suffer with yeast-related illness; if you have six or seven yes answers, you probably have a *Candida* infection; if you have eight or more yes answers, you almost certainly need medical treatment for chronic, generalized candidiasis or for unusual illnesses that occasionally mimic it. You should seek a medical diagnosis and treatment.

Have you suffered from any of the following problems:

1. Frequent infections or constant skin problems, or have you taken antibiotics (or cortisone medications) often or for long periods?
    Yes   No

2. Feelings of fatigue, being drained of energy, or drowsiness, or these symptoms on damp, muggy days or in moldy places such as a basement?
    Yes   No

3. Feelings of anxiety, irritability, or insomnia, or cravings for sugary foods, breads, or alcoholic beverages?
    Yes   No

4. Food sensitivities, allergic reactions, digestion problems, bloating, heartburn, constipation, or bad breath?
    Yes   No

5. Feeling "spacy" or "unreal," difficulty in concentrating, or being bothered by perfumes, chemical fumes, and tobacco smoke?
    Yes   No

6. Poor coordination, muscle weakness, or painful or swollen joints?

Yes   No

7. Mood swings, depression, or loss of sexual feelings?

Yes   No

8. Dry mouth or throat, nose congestion or drainage, pressure above or behind the eyes or ears, or frequent headaches?

Yes   No

9. Pains in the chest, shortness of breath, dizziness, or easy bruising?

Yes   No

10. Frustration at going from doctor to doctor, never getting your health completely well, or being told that your symptoms are "mental" or "psychological" or "psychomatic"?

Yes   No

The Vega Test Method in Naturopathic Clinics

Electro-acupuncture is a noninvasive energetic evaluation using a galvanometer. It applies biophysical techniques to traditional Asian acupuncture methods. The vegetative reflex (Vega) test method used in several naturopathic offices is the culmination of much research and was developed in Germany in 1978 by Dr. Helmut Schimmel. It requires that only one point be measured and is based on measuring against test ampoules rather than against the organ-linked point themselves.

The skin resistance on the acupuncture point is measured by producing a slight potential difference (voltage) between a tip electrode held against the point and a large hand electrode held by the patient.

The procedure measures changes in skin resistance at the acupuncture point in response to placing test substances (foods or special test ampoules) in circuit with the patient. The testing is painless, involving no needles, shocks, or scratches, and allows for the determination of specific information regarding the patient's health.

North American physicians and patients encounter more difficulty in understanding and accepting these methods as they have been educated and conditioned to view health and disease from a mainly biochemical perspective.

In a controlled, comparative study of various ways of testing for food sensitivities, Dr. Julia Tsuei compared blood, scratch, cytotoxic, food challenge, and electro-acupuncture testing. The electro-acupuncture results proved to be accurate and reproducible. The 1984 study, reported in the *American Journal of Acupuncture*, revealed that it was non-invasive but demonstrated great sensitivity.

Please see the resources at the end of this book for available diagnostic tests in your area. Diagnostic tests include tests of blood, stool, urine, saliva, and tissue or bodily fluid samples. Finding *Candida* by blood culture is considered the definitive test for systemic yeast infection.

My *Candida* Story

I have been healthy all my life. I was always determined to live a healthful, happy, fulfilling life. In 1997, I visited a naturopathic physician to make sure that I was still in good health. I had a Vega test done for food sensitivity and environmental allergies, and the *Candida* test was included. The tests revealed that I was allergic to some foods and chemicals and that my *Candida* level needed to be lowered. I realized that the antibiotics I had taken for pneumonia in 1987 had probably affected me more than I'd thought. This was confirmed by an analysis of full live blood cells and components. There is something very exciting about seeing your own live blood moving about on a video screen. As I watched the cell formations, and the naturopathic physician explained what the different blobs and squiggles meant, I felt a real sense of awe and also a little anxiety. I was looking at my life force. The lab tests usually used by medical doctors don't give the same information. They are geared to identify diseases. But the focus of the blood test in a naturopathic office is on dysfunctional and lifestyle problems. Also, most medical labs stain blood specimens to show the details of the cells, and staining kills the cells. With the darkfield microscope used in a naturopathic office and a mere one drop of blood from a fingertip, we can see the structure of live cells without stain. If a person has *Candida*, the microscope will show some fungal phenomena such as little bubbles that tend to appear around platelet clots.

The whole experience was a wakeup call for me to never take my health for granted. I started to read more seriously on natural health issues and particularly *Candida* and allergies. I worked on improving my diet and became more aware of the environmental chemicals. After six months of diligently working on my diet and taking some herbal remedies, I went back for another test and the results were very encouraging. My *Candida* level went from 7 to 2, and my allergies were improved.

In writing this story, I hope to inspire any of you who are dismayed by health problems to know that it is possible to heal yourself with help from a naturopathic physician or a natural health practitioner.

This Vega test is available at the Vancouver Naturopathic Clinic. Visit: www.vancouvernaturopathicclinic.com.

Chapter 5

Keys to a Complete Candida Cure

C andida albicans overgrowth can be healed in about two
months. Some individuals with minor problems may be cured
in as little as three to four weeks. Long-term *Candida* sufferers may
require three to four months or more of treatment, depending on the
method. Once overabundance of *Candida* yeast has been in the body,
it can easily reoccur if body systems and energy levels reach a low state
over a period of time. It is virtually impossible to wipe out all traces
of *C. albicans*; new yeast organisms enter the body easily from outside
sources in day-to-day contact with the environment. Individuals with
additional health concerns may have to repeat treatments every few
years until robust health is achieved.

To "cure" *C. albicans*, it is necessary to take care of the overgrowth
as much as possible and restore a healthful balance of friendly bacteria
within the body by consuming foods and water that do not feed the
yeast. During the healing process, body energy levels must be raised

and maintained so the body is no longer susceptible or predisposed toward an overgrowth of yeast. The body must become healthy, able to digest and assimilate foods properly, and strong enough that the yeast organisms cannot regain control because the body's restored natural defenses prevent it.

Dietary restrictions need only be placed on foods that feed yeast, weaken the body, or aggravate food sensitivities or allergies. Whether you are a vegan (one who eats no animal products, including meat, eggs, dairy, or honey), a vegetarian (one who eats no meat but enjoys dairy and eggs), a partial vegetarian (one who eats no red meat but enjoys fish and poultry), or a meat eater (one who eats all kinds of meat and other foods), dietary changes are your decision.

The goal of a *Candida* diet is mostly controlling the overgrowth of yeast while providing nutrients necessary for a healthful lifestyle. How you proceed is up to you. You do not need to restrict yourself and be fanatic about it. You can include a wide range of healthful, delicious foods.

Types of Treatment

The treatment of *Candida* overgrowth and other fungal infections is highly variable from one healthcare practitioner to another. The most important thing is to improve digestive competence and immune defense functions. The goal should never be just to kill all the *Candida* and fungi in the body. By improving digestion and the general health of the immune system, *Candida* and other fungi will not find a hospitable environment that allows them to do damage.

The single most important factor in the treatment of *Candida* overgrowth is dietary manipulation. The basis of this is that you remove the foods that *Candida* likes (essentially sugars) and therefore inhibit its growth.

Most mild and moderate cases can be treated without prescription drugs. Persistent or severe fungal infections, although responsive to the natural approach of diet changes and food supplements, might require antifungal drugs. The decision about drugs should be made after considerable discussion with one or more doctors.

The most common natural and drug treatments used by naturopaths and holistic medical doctors are described here. Most of these recommendations can be easily implemented, but it is not a good idea to self-diagnose or self-prescribe. There is no single magic pill! Arming yourself with knowledge and then seeing a healthcare practitioner for assessment and a personalized treatment regimen is best.

Holistic Diet

Food allergies can make fungal infections worse, and vice versa. A natural-healthcare practitioner can help pinpoint unsuspected food allergies that should be eliminated from the diet. Fungi thrive on sugar, especially the milk sugar lactose. Whether or not you have allergies, try to avoid foods high in sugar, fruit, fruit juice, fermented foods such as beer, wine, cheese, bread, stored grains, grain-fed animal products (red meats, especially beef and pork, animal fats, milk, and other high-fat dairy products), nuts (especially peanuts, cashews, pistachios, and dried coconuts), seeds, and refined foods. Avoid leftovers and tobacco products.

Try to eat more fish and fish oils, garlic, onions, olives, olive oil, green vegetables, herbs, spices, soy products, yogurt, psyllium, pectin, and milled (ground) flaxseed—provided you can tolerate them without symptoms. Increased intake of fiber significantly reduces the impact of mycotoxins.

Brush teeth with a natural toothpaste that includes baking soda, and use a mouthwash from a health-food store. The sweetener found in almost any type of commercial toothpaste encourages the growth of *Candida* or other fungi.

General Dietary Considerations

In the early days of *Candida* research, emphasis was placed on the need to avoid all yeasted and fermented foods. Recently, however, this has been discounted. The most current thinking suggests that for many people, eating these foods causes no problems because the *Candida* is a different strain of yeast (just as mushrooms are different from harmful fungi), and eating them will not affect the *Candida*. However, a significant number of people do have major allergic reactions to ingested or inhaled yeasts. For them, eating mushrooms or other fungi and yeasts, vinegar, miso, or other fermented foods, or inhaling spores from a moldy house, can have drastic effects on their health. In these cases the *Candida* itself is not being affected by the other fungi, but the allergic reactions can be similar to the symptoms of *Candida* overgrowth, which is presumably why the confusion arose in the first place.

The following foods are suggested for about eight weeks. After that you can add many of the restricted foods back into your diet, one at a time. Unless allergic to these foods, DO eat:

- Fresh vegetables
- Fish, poultry, and eggs (preferably free-range, and the poultry without the skin)
- Meats such as lamb, beef, wild game, eaten in moderation (once a week)
- All whole grains, including barley, millet, oats, brown rice, quinoa, and spelt
- Whole-grain muffins, tortillas, or unyeasted

- Whole-grain non-sweetened cereals
- Lentils and beans such as kidney, pinto, navy, chick, garbanzo, and peas (in soups, stews, and casseroles)
- Raw nuts and seeds (except for peanuts)
- Butter and cold-pressed oils such as flax, safflower, sesame, and olive
- Soy milk, rice dream milk, plain yogurt with *L. acidophilus* and *bifidus* (no sugar, no additives, no coloring), buttermilk, and unfermented cheeses (cream, cottage, and ricotta)
- Free-range whole eggs (preferably hard- or soft-boiled)

LIMIT your intake of the following foods:

- Sweeteners and sugars such as table sugar, fructose, corn syrup, honey, molasses, maple syrup, malt barley, and date sugar. These create overgrowth of intestinal fungi.
- Refined carbohydrates such as white flour, found in most commercial breads, pastries and pastas; short-grained or converted white rice, which usually contains yeast and sugar; and wheat, to which many people are allergic and which leads to excessive growth of fungi
- Yeast (brewer's and baking), which is found in breads, cakes, crackers, certain pastries, pretzels, and cereals
- Soy sauce and miso (except Bragg's liquid soy—non-fermented soy sauce)
- Leftover food, which tends to grow mold
- Milk and fermented cheeses, because these are converted into sugars
- Peanuts, which are sometimes contaminated with molds to which you may be allergic
- Vinegars and products containing vinegar, such as pickles, relish, sauerkraut, and most salad dressings

- Artificially sweetened drinks and food products
- Coffee (including decaffeinated) and caffeinated teas (herbal teas are usually fine)
- Alcoholic beverages, wine, beer, cola, and pop (sweetened soft drinks), because a lot of people have allergies and hypersensitivity to alcohol
- Fruit juices and dried fruit; eat a only few fruits, like apples or berries
- Mayonnaise and barbecue sauce

Other Dietary Considerations

The problem with antibiotics is that even if we don't take them orally, they are found in a lot of dairy and meat products, making our exposure to antibiotics on a daily basis almost inevitable unless we change our diet. Thankfully, today we can choose to eat organic meat and dairy products.

It is important to drink plenty of fresh water, whether bottled or filtered, mineral or reverse-osmosis water. Drink until your urine is transparent.

Digestion, food combining, and meal planning are also important to consider.

Here are some other infection-prevention tips:

- Avoid tight-fitting clothes and synthetic fabrics. Choose loose, natural fibers that breathe, like cotton underwear (white is best—there are no dyes in it).
- Avoid tight clothes like jeans, especially in the summertime.
- Choose unscented feminine hygiene products.
- Get out of wet bathing suits or workout clothes as soon as possible.

- Reduce repetitive swimming in chlorinated pools.
- Dry the vaginal area thoroughly after showering or taking baths.
- Avoid long bubble baths with perfumed or scented soaps.
- Wipe yourself from the genital area to the direction of the anus.
- Wash your underwear using unscented detergent. This will prevent allergies, skin sensitivities, and irritation in the genital area.
- Avoid vaginal deodorants and vaginal douches, as they can disturb the pH in the vagina. The pH reveals your susceptibility to or likelihood of having active infections. The average pH should be at about 6.4. When it drops to 5 or below 4, it means you are more susceptible to having infections living in your body. A higher pH of 6, 6.5, or even 7 shows that the person is not susceptible to infections, and that the infections might have cleared out of the body.
- Always urinate after sexual intercourse and wash yourself. Also, change your bed sheets after intercourse and a few times per week.
- Avoid beginning your *Candida* treatment during PMS or a week before menstual flow begins.
- Drink pure cranberry juice if you suspect an urinary infection.
- Change toothbrushes often.
- Inhale essential oils from plants such as echinacea, garlic, marigold, black walnut, and grapefruit seed through vaporization or inhalation. Also, rub a few drops of oil onto the soles of the feet, particularly the arch, so it will penetrate into the cell membranes and into the bloodstream. Massage gently twice a day. Essential oils are available in most health food and online stores.
- Read the labels when you do your grocery shopping. The starch content of whole grains gets converted into sugar. Carrots and fruit should be eaten in small quantities because they are both high in sugar.

Lifestyle

A good way to get rid of a yeast infection is to adopt new habits and keep them. It may feel a little uncomfortable in the beginning, but it will become easier, more natural, and highly rewarding with time.

Some people are more genetically prone to disease than other. However, that doesn't mean there is nothing you can do about it. You can make a difference and regain your health and energy by making positive decisions to change your lifestyle, dietary choices, and thoughts. This includes stress control, exercise, sleep optimization, and hygiene. Stress depresses your immune system. In a time of stress your body releases a hormone called cortisol, making your body defenseless against *Candida*. Stress is often a result of your own perceptions of events and the way you react to these perceptions. Changing your perceptions so that you react differently can help you control your stress level.

The daily practice of meditation can yield great rewards to the body. It helps relieves tension, promotes the healing process, and increases strength, energy and vitality. Yoga is also an excellent way to reduce stress.

Positive thinking and attitude towards life is very important. Laughter, besides being a powerful brain, respiratory, and hormonal system stimulator, is also effective at lowering blood pressure and lessening depression, and it is an excellent stress reducer. Furthermore, it decreases stress-related hormones (like cortisol, which depresses the immune system). Laughter releases hormones such as endorphins and neurotransmitters that makes us feel good.

By making a list of stress triggers and identifying their sources, you are likely to find that many of these physical, mental, and emotional triggers are completely dependent on your point of view. You can change your perspective or alter your behavior as you enter a state of stress if you wish to control it. Common life events can have a great impact on your stress level. A demanding job, a hostile boss, troubles in your marriage, debt, and so on can lead to much greater anxiety and stress. Making a list of situations that make you nervous, angry, or frustrated can help. Action is a big step in alleviating some of them and changing your perceptions of things. Just take one step at a time.

There are many researchers who claim that stress, when repressed long enough, can contribute to chronic diseases. There are various ways in which you express your stress, such as grinding teeth, overeating, undereating, rage, experiencing increased heart rate, and waking in the middle of the night.

Your thoughts create your reality. You can choose to let your thoughts get out of control or you can alter them. If you cannot change your circumstances, why not change your perspective? You can do this by converting negative self-talk into positive, identifying those thoughts when they come to your mind, and striving to find at least one aspect within the stressful situation that can be converted to positive. You can always find one.

If a person gets angry with you, remember that it's not his or her words that can harm you; it is your view of the words. You have the right to change your point of view. Nobody can take that from you. Change it and let negativity evaporate.

Sleep Optimization

Sleep is the process by which the body restores energy supplies that have been depleted through the day's activities. In sleep the body rejuvenates and repairs itself. A good night of sleep lessens anxiety and reduces stress.

○ Avoid eating heavy meals right before bedtime.
○ Avoid activities that may provoke anxiety before going to bed.

○ Make sure your bedroom is dark, comfortable, warm, and quiet.

○ Get adequate exercise (three hours before bedtime).

○ Avoid caffeine or chocolate before going to bed.

○ Take a shower or a bath just before sleeping.

You can use a dawn simulator instead of an alarm clock, which is an unnatural way of waking. One is available at www.serenityhealth.com.

Finding the right balance between working and playing is important to our mental health and overall well-being. Recreation can calm the mind and diffuse stress. For example, writing, reading, meditating, or other creative activities are emotionally, physically, and spiritually fulfilling.

Chapter 6
Candida Treatment Diets

Sometimes *Candida* overgrowth cannot be cured by diet alone, and treatment without an accompanying yeast-control diet is ineffective. Here is an example of a *Candida* treatment diet.

Treatment Diet for Regular or Severe *Candida* Control (about two months)

A gradual transition is more natural for the body and reduces the stress and anxiety that lifestyle and diet changes can sometimes create. If you are already eating a wholesome natural-food diet, it is easier to make some changes. If you are accustomed to eating the average North American diet and generally eat whatever you like at restaurants and at home, it can be difficult transition to alter your diet and restrict foods all at once.

Candida treatment change puts extra stress on the body while you are getting healthier. Extra body energy is required during treatment or change of diet. Therefore, exercise, high-nutrient foods and vitamin supplements, and extra sleep might be required.

Diet Guidelines

Enjoy: Apples, strawberries, raspberries, blueberries, blackberries, papayas, grapefruit, fresh lime or lemon juice, papaya, avocado, grapefruit. (Please see Guidelines of Foods to Enjoy.)

Try to avoid: Oranges, peaches, pineapples, mangoes, melons, grapes, cherries, bananas, plums, apricots, or fruit jams.

Try to avoid fruit that tastes too sweet, has mold on it, or is overripe. Raw fruits have live enzymes and are quickly digested when eaten alone. **Breakfast**

Drink fresh water daily upon rising

Eat the following a few times a week: 1–2 eggs, boiled, cooked, or scrambled
Whole-grain toasts
Whole-grain cereal, millet, quinoa, brown rice, or whole oats

Lunch

Eat the following a few times a week: Cooked vegetables, such as squash, broccoli, cauliflower, spaghetti squash
Soup and salad or casseroles
Vegetable juice

Omit foods that you are sensitive or allergic to.

Supper

Eat the following a few times a week: Carbohydrates (whole
grains and/or legumes)
with vegetables or proteins
(meat or dairy)
Vegetable juice

Try to avoid pork and spicy food. Avoid foods high in sugar and starch diet. Starches (carbohydrates) in breads, pasta, and potatoes are converted rapidly by our digestion process into sugar.

Try to eliminate or reduce the following foods, which tend to promote an overgrowth of *Candida* or to aggravate digestion, allergies, or sensitivities:

Alcohol
Apricots
Bacon
Baked beans
Basmati white rice
Beans (white, navy, lima, haricots, northern)
Beer
Breads made with refined grains; bagels
Cashews
Cereal (refined)
Cheeses
Cherries
Chicken (fried)
Colas
Corn
Corn chips or tortillas
Dates
Dried fruit

Eggplant
Exotic fruits
Fast food
Figs
Fish (fried)
Flour, refined
Fried foods
Fruit juices (except fresh lime or lemon)
Granola
Grapes
Greasy foods
Ham
Health bars (candy in disguise)
Hot dogs
Junk food
Macadamia nuts
Mangoes
Marinated foods
Meats (processed, fatty meats)

Melons (honeydew, cantaloupe)
Nectarines
Oily foods
Olives, green
Oranges
Peaches
Peanuts
Pickled foods
Pimentos
Pineapple
Pistachio nuts
Plums
Pork
Potatoes
Raisins
Refined foods

Rice (white)
Sausage
Shellfish (lobster,crab, shrimp, prawns,
clams, scallops, oysters, mussels, squid, octopus)
Sugar (artificial)
Tabasco sauce
Tacos
Tangerines
Vinegar
Walnuts
Wheat
Wine
Yeast, baking or nutritional

Guidelines of Foods to Enjoy (not all acceptable foods are included on this list)

Adzuki beans
Almonds (in cooking)
Artichoke hearts, cooked
Arugula
Asparagus
Avocados
Barley, cooked
Basil
Basmati rice (brown)
Bean sprouts, cooked
Beets
Black beans, cooked
Black olives, cooked
Broccoli, cooked
Brussels sprouts, cooked
Butter (dairy)
Butters (almond, filbert, pecan, sesame, sunflower, pumpkin), cooked

Cabbage, cooked or juiced
Cauliflower, cooked
Cayenne pepper
Celery
Chard, cooked
Chick peas (garbanzos), cooked
Chives, fresh, in raw or cooked foods
Cilantro, fresh, in raw or cooked foods
Club soda
Cucumbers
Cumin, cooked
Daikon (white radish)
Dulse, cooked
Eggs, cooked
Fava beans, cooked
Fennel, cooked

52

Filberts (hazelnuts), cooked
Fish (salmon, tuna, sole), cooked
Flax oil, raw only
Flax seeds
Garlic
Grapefruit (white)
Greens (kale, collard, mustard, bok choy, beet, and others), cooked
Hazelnuts, cooked
Herb teas
Herbs, raw or in cooked foods
Horseradish
Kale, cooked
Kasha (toasted buckwheat), cooked
Kelp (sea kelp), cooked
Kidney beans, cooked
Kohlrabi
Leeks, cooked
Lemon juice, fresh
Lentils, cooked
Lettuce
Lime juice, fresh
Millet, cooked
Mung beans, (cooked)
Oats (groats, whole or scotch), cooked
Oils (olive, sunflower, sesame, canola, flax, pumpkin; cold-pressed), cooked
Onions (white, yellow, red)
Paprika, cooked
Parsley
Parsnips, cooked
Peas
Pecans, cooked
Peppers
Peppers, bell (green, red, orange, yellow)

Pine nuts, cooked
Pinto beans, cooked
Pumpkin seeds, cooked
Quinoa, cooked
Radishes (red), raw
Radishes (white), raw or cooked
Red beans, cooked
Rice (long or short, brown, wild), cooked
Salmon, cooked
Scallions (green onions)
Sea kelp, cooked
Sea salt
Seaweed, cooked
Sesame salt (in cooking)
Sesame tahini, cooked
Shallots
Snow peas, cooked
Sorrel
Soy flour, cooked
Soy milk
Soy sauce (mock, Tamari), cooked
Soybeans, cooked
Spaghetti squash, cooked
Spinach

Sprouts (mung beans, alfafa sprouts), cooked
Squash (winter), cooked
Squash (yellow, summer), cooked
Sunflower seeds (use in cooking)
Tahini (sesame), cooked
Tofu, cooked
Tomato sauce, cooked
Tomatoes
Tuna, cooked
Turnips, cooked
Vegetable broth powered, cooked

Water (fresh, distilled, purified)
Water chestnuts, cooked
Wild rice, cooked
Yams (orange), cooked

Yogurt, fresh, plain, with
L. acidophilus
Zucchini

Nutritious Herbs: parsley, fennel, basil, coriander, thyme, dandelion, oregano, and mint.

Occasional Foods (a few times per week or per month)

Apple juice or cider in recipes
Barley green powder
Beef (range-fed or organic, free of petrochemicals, hormones, and fungicides)
Brazil nuts in cooking
Canned foods, cooked only
Chicken (organic or free-range is preferred)
Chili powder, cooked
Cinnamon
Curry powder, cooked
Feta cheese
Ginger, cooked
Honey (1–2 teaspoons, or minute amounts only)
Lamb, cooked
Milk
Ricotta cheese
Turkey
Turkey (free-range or organic preferred)
Veal, cooked
Watercress
Wild game meat

Constipation and Bowel problems

Many diseases generate from an unclean colon. Healthy bowel transit time should take about twelve hours. The longer food takes to process and stays in the body, the more chance there is for putrification and disease to grow over time. The colon can become a breeding ground for *Candida* and other yeasts, parasites, bacteria, and viruses.

Regular bowel movements are important. You can improve them by drinking water, increasing fiber from fruits and vegetables, exercising, or drinking tea like senna, if necessary.

Chapter 7

Is It Safe to Have Sex If You Have a Yeast Infection?

It is highly recommended that you don't have sex while you have a yeast infection. Your partner can carry the yeast for a few days and then reinfect you. It is better to wait until the infection is cured completely or under control. A yeast infection is painful, and so is sex during the infection. Some women experience a burning sensation. Arousal plays a significant part when it comes to enjoying sex. Women who are "dry" and not properly aroused by their own natural lubricants experience pain upon penetration. This can increase the chance of irritation in the vaginal area, which can lead to yeast infection. Make sure you are fully aroused before you have intercourse.

Many people do not realized that *C. albicans* can be transmitted through sexual contact. Open-mouthed kissing and oral sex can transmit *Candida* yeast.

It is preferable to have sex near the end of the time when the person with the main problem is finishing treatment. Furthermore, it is better if your partner cleans himself, including his fingers, before and after sex,.

Men can have *Candida* overgrowth just like women. The majority of *Candida* in the body resides in the intestinal tract and the colon. The average, healthy male and female have "normal" *Candida* growth in their respective bodies.

Men are susceptible to *Candida* overgrowth from antibiotics, stress, steroids, poor diet, drugs, alcohol, genetic predispositions, hydrochloric acid deficiency, and metal toxicity from mercury, copper, iron, etc. A difference between men's and women's yeast infection is that men cannot get those annoying vaginal yeast infections that are the "red flag" of yeast overgrowth in women. However, they can get penile yeast infections or experience many other symptoms that may never be associated with their *Candida* overgrowth!

Men can have yeast overgrowth in their urinary systems and can implant yeast into a woman's vaginal area during intercourse or into the mouth during oral sex.

The treatment of men's yeast infections follows similar methods for that of women. Most medication and treatment for yeast overgrowth is targeted at women. This infection is a result of the overgrowth of *Candida* yeast on the surface of the skin. It is usually typified by symptoms. The fungus thrives in areas of the skin that are moist and hot. This makes the infection more common in summer and in countries with warm weather. The groin and genitals are mostly affected, although infection has also been found on the mouth. Symptoms could be as simple as itching and general discomfort. Other symptoms are dry, whitish skin and penile discharge in more severe cases.

A man can be infected through sexual relationship with a woman who has *Candida* overgrowth. Men with diabetes, which causes excess body sugar, are also prone to the disease. Some of the other causes include diet, prolonged use of antibiotics, and the wearing of tight clothing.

There are several over-the-counter medications that give relief to mild cases of yeast infections. The only problem is that the infection tends to reoccur. Effective treatment of male yeast infection involves a more holistic approach. Men with severe or recurring symptoms have to do more than just rubbing one or the other cream on the affected areas of their skin. A change of lifestyle is required to get rid of yeast infection.

Natural treatment of male yeast infection has been found to be effective. This treatment involves the use of natural substances that do not have any side effects. Some men have found that ginger is one of the best natural antibiotics and has proven to be effective against the condition. Apple cider vinegar diluted in water and used to wash the affected area a couple of times a day is also good. Treatment of male yeast infection also includes a change in diet, including the elimination of sugary foods that encourage fungal growth, and the consumption of foods rich in fiber and vitamins that will enhance the body's immunity.

Food Influences

"A night out with the boys" can easily encourage *Candida* overgrowth. High-carbohydrate foods like pasta, French fries, and bread, along with beer, can encourage *Candida* growth. The maltose level in beer can feed the pre-existing yeast colonies in the intestinal tract and make them spread. Beer might also aggravate nail fungus, jock itch, and skin rashes.

Hormones

While men are not estrogen-dominated like women—and not prone to yeast problems due to spikes in estrogen that occur during a menstrual cycle—as men get older, their ratio of estrogen to testosterone rises. This change subjects a man to yeast overgrowth and prostate difficulties. Yeast can and does invade the prostate, causing infections that will not resolve with antibiotics. In fact, when treated with antibiotics, the infections typically return.

Menopause and Men

"Andropause" is that time in a man's life when his testosterone levels begin to drop. This occurs at any time after the age of forty in the United States and after the age of fifty in Europe. As testosterone and DHEA drop, estrogens tend to rise. The stress hormone cortisol also tends to rise as men and women age. Cortisol further blocks the effects of testosterone and DHEA and can cause many of the signs and symptoms of "aging." This same hormone pattern encourages the overgrowth of *Candida*.

Candida Symptoms in Men

- Burning sensation when urinating
- Pain during sexual intercourse
- Rash (along the shaft or on the tip of the penis)
- Burning sensation of the infected area
- Slight swelling

- Light discharge
- Pain during ejaculation
- Burning after ejaculation or urinating
- Low sperm count or semen volume
- Gas, bloating, or belching
- Poor digestion
- Constipation or diarrhea
- Loss of sex drive
- Mild to severe erectile dysfunction
- Loss of muscle tone or mass
- Loss of strength
- Rectal itch
- Itchy mouth or tongue
- White coating on tongue
- Thrush of the mouth
- Painful tongue
- Sore throat
- Prostate cancer or enlarged prostate
- Dry skin or skin rashes
- Craving for sweets and starches
- Depression or moodiness
- Insomnia despite exhaustion
- Flu-like symptoms
- Hip, groin, or lower back pain
- Sore feet or painful heels
- Allergies to yeast, vinegar, or alcohol
- Sleepiness after meals
- Intolerance or sensitivity to alcohol
- Hay fever
- Asthma
- Chronic sinus infections or congestion

Yeast Infection in Men

These infections are likely to occur at the end of the penis, under the foreskin. A male yeast infection in the penis is known as balanitis. Men with a foreskin are more prone to male yeast infections because the warmth and moisture underneath the skin encourages the growth of fungi.

A male yeast infection is not classified as a sexually transmitted infection because many men already have small amounts of the *Candida* fungus living on the penis. People who have never been sexually active can still suffer from yeast infections for the reasons stated earlier in this book. *Candida* likes warm and moist skin. If the skin of your genitals is already irritated by perfumes in soaps or shower gels, if you are careless about drying yourself after washing, or if you have diabetes that is uncontrolled (perhaps because you are unaware you have diabetes), *Candida* is more likely to multiply. When it does, you may begin to notice symptoms as a male yeast infection develops.

Most Common Male Yeast Infection (Balanitis) Symptoms

- Irritation and soreness of the head of the penis
- Severe itching on the head of the penis
- White, clumpy discharge
- Redness on the head of the penis
- Small blisters on the head of the penis

Chapter 8
Thrush

Thrush is a yeast infection of the mouth, throat, or tongue. Most typically caused by *C. albicans*, it can affect different part of the body such as the skin, genitals, and digestive tract. It often occurs in people whose immune system is compromised. Drugs currently on the market do not tackle the root of the problem, which is your body's ability to naturally control the thrush. Under normal conditions, *Candida* yeast is typically present in the human body. In a healthy person, the immune system and other naturally occurring microorganisms keep *Candida* in check or under control.

Symptoms of thrush may include severe itching, burning and soreness, sore tongue, canker sores, and heartburn. Many sufferers have a white- or yellowish-coated tongue. This is thrush, oral candidasis, or oropharyngeal candidasis. It can happen in women, men, and children. To completely cure the thrush, we need to bring our bodies back into balance and be healthy again.

Lozenges (pastilles) are sometimes used as an alternative treatment to oral rinses like nystatin (Nilstat, Mycostatin, Bio-Statin, and Nystex) and clotrimazole (Mycelex). Lozenges are limited to direct contact with the yeast cells in the mouth, however, and thus do not solve the real cause of the problem. They are aimed at alleviating the symptoms while ignoring the true cause of the illness.

Immediately after sexual intercourse, gargle with antibacterial mouthwash or sea-salt water.

The most common symptoms of a male oral yeast infection are white spots in the mouth and on the tongue that do not wipe off and are painful, especially when eating and drinking. Men who get yeast infections invariably believe it's sexually transmitted. Although this is possible, most experts say that male yeast infections aren't usually the result of unprotected sex and often develop in men who aren't sexually active. However, if you have a regular female partner, it is quite likely that she will also be carrying *Candida* in her vagina.

So What Do I Do?

If you chronically get vaginal yeast infections after intercourse, begin using condoms to stop the flow of yeast that might be coming from your partner to you. That's the first important step.

Ask your partner to take the *Candida* questionnaire on the website at http://www.health-truth.com/185.php. Ask him to be tested for yeast overgrowth by a practitioner who is familiar with the subject. Make sure the stool, urine, and blood tests are done. If he has high scores on the questionnaire but the tests come out negative, assume the tests missed it and seek treatment or better tests.

If necessary, you can ask your partner to be tested for hormones to see if they are imbalanced in the manner described here, which could encourage yeast overgrowth. If he has yeast overgrowth, ask him to get treated fully. Make sure the treatment will keep the yeast overgrowth under control in his urinary tract, intestinal tract, and systemically.

Make sure this program involves balancing the intestinal flora and healing the gut lining. The program should address the flora after the yeast is gone. Friendly bacteria cannot grow in an intestine that is full of yeast.

Chapter 9

Natural Antifungal Treatments

The major disadvantage of drug therapy is the cost, but significant side effects can also be a problem with any non-natural treatments. Natural therapies, for the most part, are safe. They involve diet changes and the use of one or a combination of the following supplement options. A list of the more prominent antifungal and antibacterial remedies includes berberine, goldenseal (a source of berberine), caprylic acid, oil of oregano, black walnut, cat's claw, pau d'arco, and olive-leaf extract.

Exercise is an effective antifungal therapy because *Candida* and fungi do not thrive in a high-oxygen environment. A higher oxygen level can be created in the body by regular exercise. For those who can participate in physical activity, exercise is beneficial.

Berberine is an alkaloid found in herbs such as goldenseal, barberry, and Oregon grape. It fights *Candida* and parasites (especially amoeba) overgrowth and normalizes intestinal flora. Berberine stimulates the immune system, soothes inflamed mucus membranes, and helps diarrhea and other gastrointestinal symptoms. It is very well tolerated and generally associated with no side effects.

Betaine and pepsin hydrochloride, as well as other stomach acidifiers like glutamic acid and stomach bitters, dissolve *Candida* and fungi in the stomach. Antacids and acid-suppressing drugs like cimetidine and ranitidine lead to fungal infections because they eliminate the fungal-protective effect of hydrochloric acid. Excess acid, however, can cause severe heartburn and lead to gastritis or peptic ulcer disease. The need for acid supplementation should be determined by tests ordered by a natural healthcare practitioner. One of the tests is the comprehensive stool and digestive analysis.

Biotin is a B-complex vitamin that is important particularly for the health of the hair, skin, and nails. It inhibits the conversion of the benign yeast form of *Candida* into the invasive mycelial form. The usual effective therapeutic dose in adults is 1 milligram or more daily. *Lactobacillus acidophilus* and other good bacteria produce most of our B vitamins, including biotin. However, a supplement might be necessary for healing the overgrowth of *C. albicans*.

Caprylic acid is a naturally occurring antifungal fatty acid (from coconut oil) and works primarily at the level of the gastrointestinal tract. It is comparable in its antifungal activity to the prescription drug nystatin. It only has weak systemic antifungal properties.

Citrus-seed extracts (paracan 144, paramicrocidin, citricidal) are advocated by several well-known holistic doctors. These products are as effective as nystatin and caprylic acid in the treatment of gut-fungus overgrowth. Parasites like giardia and blastocystis hominis are effectively treated by citrus-seed extracts. Take in warm water, one hour or more before or after meals or starches to avoid stomach upset.

Cloves and clove tea have a similar effect to pau d'arco and can be used effectively against any fungal or parasitic infestation.

Coenzyme Q10 is an antioxidant normally found in the body and is involved in optimizing the effects of oxygen in the body. CoQ10 (ubiquinone) has been well documented in helping the many symptoms of chronic fatigue syndrome, angina pectoris, and high blood pressure. It has no side effects or significant toxicity.

Colloidal silver is a broad-spectrum antifungal product gaining widespread use with alternative healthcare practitioners due to its antiviral and antibacterial properties. Silver in a colloidal form is non-toxic to human cells. It works by disabling enzyme systems found in bacteria, viruses, and fungi.

Dioxychlor, aerobic oxygen, bioxy cleanse, and other oral forms of oxygen work based on the ability to harm fungi by increasing oxygen in the body. They may not be as effective as intravenous ozone or hydrogen peroxide therapy, but case histories indicate a substantial benefit and symptom reversal in many cases.

Fish and fish oils (omega-3- and omega-6-EPA fatty acids) have been demonstrated to substantially reduce the mortality rate from atherosclerosis. Fish oils and other fatty acids have strong antifungal properties. Some individuals benefit a great deal from supplementing their diets with fish like salmon and tuna.

Flaxseed oil is a good source of omega-3- and omega-6-EPA fatty acids. Evening primrose oil, borage oil, and black currant seed oil are excellent sources of omega-6-EPA fatty acids. All are antifungal.

Grapefruit-seed extract was discovered to have antimicrobial and antibacterial activity It is sometimes referred to as citrus-seed extract. It is made by first converting grapefruit seeds and pulp into a very acidic liquid. The liquid is loaded with polyphenolic compounds, including quercitin, helperidin, campherol glycoside, neohelperidin, naringing, apigenin, rutinoside, poncirin, and others. The final product is bitter and acidic.

Garlic and onions have been used for thousands of years as antibiotic, antifungal, and health-enhancing foods. They have a significant role to play in the prevention and treatment of heart disease and cancer. Garlic and onions are mainstays of any effective natural antifungal program. Both are potent in lowering cholesterol and triglycerides. For those who cannot tolerate the taste or odor caused by garlic, garlic oil capsules or combinations of garlic and parsley are good substitutes. Garlic strengthens the immune system. Use garlic as soon as you feel any symptoms of *Candida* overgrowth. A substitute to garlic can be shallots or onions. Personally, garlic added to my food several times a week has worked like a miracle for me to prevent the overgrowth of *Candida*. Garlic can help fight yeast infections both externally and internally. If eaten raw, it needs to be chopped to activate its powerful ingredients. Garlic lowers blood pressure, so if you suffer from low blood pressure, do not consume garlic excessively. If you are on anticoagulants, consult your doctor before taking garlic therapeutically.

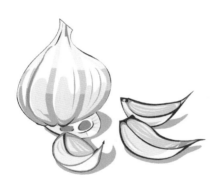

Ginger tea is the hot beverage of choice to soothe inflammation in the gastrointestinal tract caused by *Candida* or fungal overgrowth, as well as to help repair inflamed tissues.

Green food supplements are effective against *Candida* overgrowth and fungi primarily because of their immune system–boosting properties. High chlorophyll content prevents the spread of fungal or bacterial infection and promotes the growth of friendly colonic bacteria. Some of the green foods with well documented benefits are barley greens, chlorella, spirulina, blue-green algae, and green kamut. High-quality popular brands blended with synergistic herbs and plant enzymes are Greens Plus (Supplements Plus) and Green Life (Bioquest). These are available in powder form for better absorption and are often prescribed for boosting energy and immunity.

Homeopathic remedies (aquaflora, candex, and others) contain very diluted, almost imperceptible amounts of *C. albicans* and other fungi. Unlike herbal, vitamin, mineral, enzyme, and prescription medicine antifungals, homeopathic remedies for fungi have little scientific documentation to support their use. It is unknown how many people suffering from fungal infections clear the infection or hypersensitivity with these products. The *Candida* syndrome is linked to perhaps thousands of different fungi or strains of *Candida*; the *C. albicans* homeopathic dilutions might not be specific enough for many victims of fungal infection or hypersensitivity. Thousands of patients and homeopathic doctors, however, have claimed excellent results in reversing signs and symptoms of chronic fungal problems with homeopathic remedies. These products are harmless and, under supervision of a qualified homeopathic doctor, may make a big difference for certain individuals.

Kelp, dulse, and seaweeds are exceptionally good antifungal whole foods. They are rich in iodine and selenium, two minerals known for their ability to inactivate fungi. Before antifungal drugs, iodine was the main effective remedy against *Candida* and fungi.

Lactobacillus acidophilus **and** *bifidus* are friendly bacteria, normal inhibitants of the gastrointestinal tract. Their presence is one of the body's natural defenses against fungal invasion. Yogurt and other cultured dairy products are good dietary sources; these bacteria can also be obtained from non-dairy sources, in powder or encapsulated forms. They are highly recommended if prescription antibiotics are used to treat bacterial infections.

L-cysteine is an amino acid with a detoxifying effect. It can chelate many toxins related to fungal and *Candida* overgrowth.

Olive oil, castor bean oil, and oregano oil are antifungal and have no known side effects except diarrhea if used in excessively large amounts. Some supplement companies manufacture capsules containing these extracts.

Other immune-system boosters reported to benefit the treatment of fungal infections include ashwaganda, astragalus, barley sprouts, chaparral, licorice root, myrrh, thymus gland extract, safflower oil, and eucalyptus oil. Blends of antifungals are found in easily tolerated Candida-zyme and Candida Cleanse.

Liver-cleansing herbs include dandelion, burdock, and milk thistle. Herbal supplements to cleanse and eliminate toxins are available at www.blessedherbs.com. Nature's Secret/Irwin Naturals Ultimate Cleanse milk thistle is available at www.naturessecret.com.

Metal cleanse. Mercury dental fillings might create health problems, yeast infections among them. Chemical and toxic metal build-up inside the body can also lead to hormonal imbalance and weakening of the immune system. There might be heavy metals (lead, silver, mercury) coming from food, the air we breathe, medicines, and dental fillings. For individuals who suffer from acute metal toxicity, urine, blood, and stool analyses have shown to be accurate. However, for the vast majority of those with *Candida* overgrowth who have mild to moderate heavy-metal problems, these tests are mostly inconclusive. Kinesiology tests and electrical readouts might be more accurate. Chelation therapy is also available. Please contact your local naturopaths or integrative MDs. You can also take foot detoxification baths (heavy metals are eliminated through the pores of your feet). Furthermore, Lugol's iodine foot rub might be therapeutic.

Lugols iodine foot rub. Rub 2-4 drops of Lugol's iodine on your feet. This will enhance heavy-metal detoxification. Keep applying the iodine to your feet for several days. This is a powerful yet inexpensive detoxification process for heavy metals that you can do in the privacy of your own home. Lugol's iodine can be ordered online at www.amazon.com or www.finlandiapharmacyonline.com.

Oxygen therapies (ozone, hydrogen peroxide, dioxychlor, and coenzyme Q10) are extremely effective natural antifungal treatments, the treatment of choice in chronic, intractable cases of systemic fungal infections, and, for some people, superior to all prescription antifungal drugs. Visiting your natural healthcare practitioner for personalized advice on oxygen treatments is best.

Pau d'arco (la pacho or taheebo) is an effective antifungal remedy, available in loose tea form or as a tincture.

Peppermint oil (enteric-coated) is used as an antispasmodic remedy in the treatment of irritable bowel syndrome; it happens to be anticandidal and antifungal as well.

Tea tree oil (*Melaleuca alternifolia*) is a broad-spectrum antiseptic (fungi, bacteria, parasites) traditionally used as an effective remedy against all types of *Candida* infections.

Vitamin B6 is a water-soluble vitamin consisting of three related compounds: pyridoxine, pyridoxal, and pyridoxamine. It is an important adjunctive therapy for *Candida* problems, especially in women with history of birth-control pill usage. Vitamin B6 is found in a large number of healthful foods, including legumes, seeds, green leafy vegetables, avocados, soybeans, and walnuts. Vitamin B6 assists in red blood cell regeneration and helps regulate protein, fat, and carbohydrate utilization.

Specific Anti-Yeast Supplements

1. Olive leaf extract or oregano oil (for no more than two weeks). When adding olive leaf extract or oregano oil along with garlic to your diet, use 1 part of oil of oregano to 5–10 parts olive oil. A few drops of oregano are all you need; oregano oil is very potent. You can use oil of oregano to blend salads. Available at www. mothernature.com.

2. Caprylic acid or calcium-magnesium caprylate. For seven days you can take up to 500 mg daily.

3. SF-722 by Thorne Research (Healthy Gut and Vaginal Flora). The active ingredient 10-undecenoic acid from the castor bean has been proven to be effective against all types of *Candida* infections. Please visit www.thorne.com. Also available at www.amazon.com.

4. Candigest in capsules. This supplement will eradicate most systemic yeast infection with all its associated symptoms in less than thirty days. Candigest Plus is available at http://www. imunecare.co.uk.

5. CandiZyme by Renew Life. These enzymes can help you with *Candida* overgrowth. There is also a Candida Solution kit available at www.renewlife.com.

Natural Products to Eliminate Symptoms in Twelve Hours

Garlic. Eat crushed, raw garlic in your food several times a day. For thrush and sore tongue, suck a very small piece of garlic clove in your mouth or place it directly on the sore area of the tongue. If you can tolerate it, crush it with your teeth. The inulin found in garlic is a type of fiber that the good intestinal bacterium loves. It can quickly and effectively fight yeast infection and eradicate all the symptoms associated with it. (Do not use garlic on genitals.)

Gentian violet. Beside its ability to be messy and stain clothes, this dark purple dye was proven to be effective. However, some people might experience tingles or mild skin irritation. Soak a tampon in about one tablespoon of gentian violet, insert into the vagina, and leave it for several hours. Use a tampon with a plastic applicator, and wear gloves and black underwear. To avoid stains, use black towels to protect your floor and counter before use. Gentian violet might be available in a pharmacy or drugstore. Use this method only if necessary and for quick relief. For external use only.

Yogurt (plain, no coloring, additives, fruit or sugar). Apply to the skin with a spatula or finger and leave for about one hour. You will feel great relief with a cooling and soothing sensation from this simple treatment. This can also be effective for men. Men should also apply tea tree oil, calendula cream, or pure aloe vera gel to the affected area.

Tea tree oil is a powerful antifungal agent and is effective on skin. It reduces redness and rejuvenates. Besides being antibacterial, it is antiviral and antiseptic. Especially for sensitive skin, it's important not to use a 100 percent pure concentration of tea tree oil. The maximum concentration recommended is 20 percent tea tree oil, diluted with jojoba oil. Pure certified organic tea tree oil can be available in a health-food store or can be ordered online at http://mothernature.com.

Chapter 10
Drugs for Selected Individuals

S ome fungal or *Candida* infections do not respond to the natural approach. This could either be because (1) the individual finds it difficult or impossible to make the diet changes or tolerate the supplements or (2) the infection is too longstanding and entrenched in many different organs and tissues in the body. Some patients who have treated their *Candida* overgrowth for a year or longer without much benefit could certainly give the drug approach some consideration. Careful use of antifungal drugs might be a very effective option. Of course, since all these drugs require a prescription, they must be monitored for potential side effects on a regular basis. Drugs such as ketoconazole, for example, although generally well tolerated, can occasionally adversely affect liver function. Regular lab tests should be done in order to observe any abnormalities and thereby prevent organ damage.

Commonly Prescribed Drugs

Drugs, creams, and lotions are designed to tackle the symptoms of yeast infections, not the real cause. Most conventional treatments for *Candida* infection work as a temporary solution but fail to work in the long run.

The most commonly prescribed drugs for *Candida* and fungal infections are: amphotericin B (Fungizone), aspirin, caspofungin (Cancidas), colchicine, fluconazole (Diflucan), flucytosine (5-F), griseofulvin, Gynazole, itraconazole (Sporanox), ketoconazole (Nizoral), miconazole (Monistat), nystatin (Nilstat), Terazol, terbinafine (Lamisil), and voriconazole (Vfend).

Canesten and Monistat are available without a prescription. Doctors and pharmacists often recommend Canesten in vaginal tablets or cream in a one-, three-, or six-day treatment. Those treatments might be useful for emergency relief or to reduce inflammation. However, they do not treat the real causes of the yeast infections.

The Side Effects of Canesten (Most popular and advertised)

Many medications cause side effects that can be mild or severe, temporary or permanent. The side effects listed below are not experienced by everyone but have been reported by some people taking this medication:

- Abdominal bloating, upset stomach
- Burning sensation
- Stomach cramping and pain
- Irritation, reaction to the medication, intolerance
- Itching

- Rash, redness, swelling
- Fever, chills, vomiting

Although most of the following side effects don't happen very often, they could lead to serious problems:

- Hives
- Peeling
- Vaginal bleeding
- Blistering

Chapter 11
Rotating Treatments

One problem associated with treatments for *Candida* overgrowth is the eventual resistance to the therapy in use. Fungi adapt to natural as well as drug remedies if used for extended periods of time. There is even evidence that fungi can grow and spread more rapidly on antifungal drugs after exposure for extended periods. Patients on prescription drugs such as nystatin often develop sensitivity to the drug when used in high doses for months at a time. If one rotates an antifungal remedy, *Candida* and other fungi are less likely to develop resistance, and the patient is less likely to develop an allergy or hypersensivity to that remedy.

The following food recommendations should be helpful against *Candida* overgrowth.

- All vegetables, including leafy greens, beet tops, broccoli, cabbage, celery, chlorophyll, kale, onions, rutabaga, turnips, and wheatgrass

- Some fruit juices and a diet high in complex carbohydrates, protein, and fiber
- Herbs including barberry bark, black walnut, dong quai, garlic, grapefruit-seed extract, pau d'arco, primrose oil, and red clover
- Yogurt
- Reduced intake of alcohol, butter, cheeses in all forms, chocolate, citrus and dried fruits, fermented foods, glutens, ham, honey, nut, pickles, soy/tamari sauces, sugar, and yeast products

Important nutrients include:

- Essential fatty acids (found in black currant–seed oil and flax-seed oil)
- Yogurt with *L. acidophilus* or *bio-bifidus*
- Caprylic acid
- Garlic
- Quercetin
- Bromelain
- Vitamin B complex
- Vitamin B12
- Calcium, magnesium, vitamin D
- Coenzyme Q10
- Multivitamin and mineral complex with vitamin A
- Epresat liquid multivitamins and herbal formulas
- Selenium
- Grapefruit-seed extract
- Vitamin C
- Herbs pau d'arco, clove tea

The term *probiotic* means "for life" in ancient Greek. Probiotics are friendly bacteria that are cultured in a laboratory and are aimed at rebalancing the flora in your digestive system. The vast majority of industrial yogurts are heated. The heating process gives yogurt longer shelf life but destroys all the friendly bacteria. The majority of brands that carry the label "made with active cultures" are misleading; all yogurts are made with active cultures, but most of them contain little to no bacteria due to the heating process. Probiotics Bio-K is probably one of the best in the market. It can be found in health-food stores like Whole Foods Market or online at www.mothernature.com. Take *Lactobacillus acidophilus/bifidus* 2 grams of *powder* three times daily between meals or Probiotics Bio-K *liquid* (dairy, soy, or rice) in one small bottle of 98g daily.

I find that liquid or powder forms are easier to digest. Also, you can open the capsules and put them in water or food, if you order capsules. If you prefer tablets, there is a Probiotic (four billion) that you can order online at www.achilleshealthmart.com.

Other remedies you might try include:

- Arginine (an amino acid), 3 grams nightly (for one month only)
- Olive oil (cold-pressed organic), 1 teaspoon daily
- Raw garlic, 1 clove daily, chopped finely in food or taken in capsule form
- Homeopathic Candida 30x, 5 drops daily
- Caprylic acid (brand names include Caprystatin, Caprycin, and Candistat-300); dosage depends on the brand selected
- Citricidal (grapefruit-seed extract), 10 drops or 1 tablet or capsule daily

Chapter 12

Where to Find Candida Overgrowth Treatments

Natural *Candida* overgrowth treatments and food remedies can be purchased at most health-food stores. Garlic and food treatments are more beneficial if they are organic. Most natural herbal treatments and special nonprescription remedies are available from a holistic pharmacy or naturopathic physician. However, some physicians will only sell treatments to their own patients. Prescription drugs, of course, must be prescribed by a medical doctor and purchased at a pharmacy.

Naturopathic doctors and nutritionists are most eager to help you.

Herbs and Foods for Fighting Candida Overgrowth

Many whole foods and herbs are effective treatments against *Candida* and other fungal infections. Whenever possible, use whole-food concentrates rather than single-nutrient tablets or capsules. Whole foods contain phytochemicals, linked to the prevention and treatment of major degenerative diseases such as heart disease, stroke, high blood blessure, and cancer. The only way to get these phytochemicals is from eating whole foods or live whole food concentrates.

Some of the best-known phytochemicals are:

- **Indoles and isothiocyanantes**, found in cruciferous vegetables like broccoli, Brussels sprouts, cabbage, cauliflower, kale, bok choy, rutabaga, and turnips. They help protect against colon cancer. Evidence is mounting that these phytochemicals also help in the prevention and treatment of other cancers, most notably breast cancer. All are antifungal.
- **Isoflavones** such as genistein, found in soybean products like soy milk. Isoflavones offset the negative effects of excessive estrogen in breast and ovarian cancer. They are antifungal.
- **Limonene**, found in citrus fruits, which produce enzymes that eliminate cancer-causing substances from the body. Citrus fruits are known for their high content of vitamin C and bioflavonoids, vital for optimal immune system function.
- **Phytosterols**, found in soybeans, which can lower the absorption of cholesterol from the diet and prevent colon cancer.
- **Kelp, dulse, bladderwrack, and other seaweeds** are exceptionally good antifungal whole foods. They are rich in iodine and selenium, minerals known for their ability to inactivate fungi.
- **Other foods** include garlic, lemon juice, aloe vera, wheatgrass, barley-green juice, cloves, onions, cayenne pepper, pau d'arco, and parsley.

It is better not to use these food remedies if you are sensitive or allergic to them. It is also imperative to not take too many healing herbs, foods, and treatments at once. Some people can make themselves ill by overtreating *Candida* overgrowth.

Healthy Balance between Alkaline and Acid

For the human body to function at its best, it has to have an internal chemistry balance of alkaline with a pH of 7.0–8.0. A diseased cell has an alkaline of below 7.0. The typical Western diet consists mainly of highly acidic products such as dairy, meat, and artificial sweeteners, while it is deprived of alkaline-producing foods such as vegetables and fruits.

Stress and negative thoughts also cause an acidic environment in the body.

Consuming About 75 Percent Raw Food

Raw food is live and uncooked, plant-based, and preferably organic. It is not necessary to calculate percentages. Simply eat one cooked meal per day and make sure the rest of the food you consume is raw. Raw foods have high quantities of enzymes and are digested more effectively. A raw-food diet consists of fresh, low-sugar vegetables, seeds, beans, seaweeds, nust and grains, and freshly made vegetable juices. This diet increases energy, accelerates the healing process, rebuilds healthy tissue, and invigorates our bodies.

Raw food is basically alkalizing and more beneficial. Cooking often destroys vitamins and minerals, fiber and enzymes. Enzymes are partly responsible for getting rid of toxic waste, purifying the blood and digesting food.

Your Doctor's Role during Treatment

Most people with *Candida* or fungal overgrowth or sensitivity can get significant help from a professional naturopath or nutritionist. Naturopathy is a system of treating disease that avoids drugs and surgery and emphasizes the use of natural agents. Complicated or more severe cases may need the help of a medical doctor and prescribed drugs.

Chapter 13
Candida and Allergies

It is true that many people with *Candida* problems have concurrent allergic problems. This is probably related to the leaky gut syndrome and the fact that their immune systems are weakened by prolonged battle with the *Candida* and the stresses of living with this type of illness.

Candida overgrowth can cause food intolerance and environmental sensitivities. As toxins enter the bloodstream as an adverse reaction to these pollutants, they can cause food allergies, food intolerance, and environmental sensitivities that in the long run can manifest into more serious conditions that weaken the immune system.

As *Candida* overgrows, it develops legs called rhizoids that penetrate the gut wall, causing inflammation and physical damage. Combined with impaired biochemical processes, this can result in a condition called leaky gut syndrome. From here *Candida* enters the bloodstream and invades all areas in the body where the immunity is weak. Leaky gut syndrome can eventually lead to bowel disorders, food sensitivities, severe allergies, and even asthma. Leaky gut syndrome is responsible for some of the symptoms of chronic *Candida* infection such as bloating, pain, heartburn, gas, constant hunger, hemorrhoids, constipation, and liver dysfunction.

It is preferable that you attend a practitioner who is trained in one of the several methods of clinical allergy testing such as Vega or kinesiology. Such a practitioner can help you formulate a diet to avoid your particular allergens and will often provide remedies to desensitize you to your allergens.

Substitutes for *Candida*-Aggravating Foods

Dairy products, especially cow's milk, are probably one of the most notorious causes of allergies. They are loaded with hormones given to the animals in order to increase their milk production. Dairy products are also filled with antibiotics that affect our bodies and hormonal balance.

It is better to avoid cow's milk, most cheeses, and products that contain lactose, milk proteins, or dry skim-milk powder. There are many substitutes now available in health-food stores. Soya products like soy milk—for example, Silk soy beverage—can serve as an alternative. Another is nut and seed milk, such as almond milk. If you are not lactose intolerant, goat and sheep milk are also good alternatives to cow's milk.

Another food that some people might be allergic to is white sugar. Processed sugar is sugar cane that has been stripped of its essential fiber and nutrients. It has no protein and no calcium. There are various terms for sugar, including the more common ones like sucrose, fructose, maltose, lactose, glycogen, glucose, mannitol, sorbitol, galactose, monosaccharide, and polysaccharide.

Honey or stevia are good substitutes for sugar. Once your *Candida* overgrowth is under control, you can slowly introduce unrefined cane sugar into your diet in moderation.

White flour, white rice, and refined, puffed, or extruded grains (including any type of cereal, puffed rice, and bran) should be avoided. These ingredients, once refined, are peeled out of their precious and nutritious pulp which is filled with vitamins and minerals. Substitutes might be brown rice, preferably organic, and whole rye.

Substitutes for gluten grains like rye, wheat, barley, bran, and corn include whole non-gluten grains like amaranth, quinoa, and buckwheat.

Hydrogenated and partly hydrogenated oils are changed molecular oils (hydrogenation keeps oils and fats from going rancid). They are found in margarine, donuts, muffins, salad dressing, candy, cakes, soups, breads, fried foods, mayonnaise, hydrogenated and partly hydrogenated soybean oil, vegetable oil, and in most processed foods. A good substitute is pure extra-virgin olive oil.

Red meat like beef and pork contains harmful toxins such as uric acid and steroids. Its hard-to-digest protein causes lots of digestion problems and allergies. Red meat also contains antibiotics, harmful hormones, and diseases the animal may have had. Substitutes include organic red meat, organic chicken, and fish like salmon and tuna.

Many people are allergic to the gluten found in wheat products like flour, pasta, and bread, such as baker's yeast, brewer's yeast, engevita, torula and other nutritional yeast, and all baked goods raised with yeast such as breads, rolls, crackers, bagels, and pastries. Those foods should be avoided if possible.

Vinegar is made with yeast culture and should be avoided during *Candida* treatment or if you are allergic to vinegar. That includes white vinegar, red wine vinegar, balsamic vinegar, commercial salad dressing, ketchup, steak sauce, soy sauce, pickles, and relishes. These foods can be reintroduced later. Substitutes include organic apple cider vinegar (Bragg's), but no more than one tablespoon a day

Food Allergens

Food allergies are often common in patients with yeast infections. Some individuals have a weakened immune system as a direct result of consuming foods that their immune system regards as allergens. Eliminating those foods can improve or clear *Candida* infections. Common foods that trigger an allergic reaction include gluten grains, wheat, corn, peanuts, dairy, soy products, and eggs.

There are two kinds of allergic reactions to food:

1. Delayed reactions make up 90 percent of the food allergies. The reaction can occur up to four days after the specific food was ingested.
2. Immediate reactions make up 10 percent of allergies, when the allergic reaction occurs from seconds to a few hours after the specific food was ingested

There are three common tests that can be used to detect allergies: the Vega test, RAST (radio allegro sorbent test), and the ELISA (enzyme-linked-immuno sorbent assay). Those tests can detect up to 100 foods.

If you prefer a simple way of treating food allergies, avoid allergenic foods for about eight weeks until symptoms are alleviated.

A good source to learn more about food allergies is the book *Allergies: Disease in Disguise*, by Carolee Bateson-Koch, DC, ND.

You Are What You Eat?

While some say you are what you eat, I say you are what you digest. Optimal digestion is far more important than the quality of food. The way you combine the food you eat and the environment you choose for eating are also important factors for the digestion process.

A good combination is to eat raw or cooked vegetables with concentrated foods such as meat, eggs, cheese, grains, legumes, nuts, and starches.

Don't exercise immediately after you have finished a meal. The body rushes the blood toward your muscles from your digestive system. As a result, your digestive system stops digesting until you stop your activity.

Find the least distracting and least noisy place to eat your meals. When you eat, try to focus on your meal and savor it. It is also important to not be in a state of stress or be upset when you eat.

Chapter 14
Regulation of Treatment

Some people need stronger treatment; some need it for longer periods of time. Sometimes a different treatment is required. Sometimes after one type of treatment, a different follow-up treatment is a good idea. Some people require a rotation of treatments—a different remedy each day for four days or so, then repeated. Sometimes multiple treatments of two or more remedies are most effective. Your doctor can help you determine what works best for you.

Some individuals respond well to prescription drugs, while others require natural treatment. Some patients deal with the treatment process easily; the majority have side effects that make the treatment uncomfortable and even agonizing for a few.

Some people are not always told by their doctors that *Candida* overgrowth symptoms will usually get worse during treatment before they get better. As the yeast overgrowth dies off, the body is filled with ins. This weakens the entire body, making all symptoms worse or a while. This is one reason for side effects. Another is that your "treatment" may not be right for you. Some people with allergy problems or chronic fatigue syndrome or low blood sugar cannot tolerate nystatin, ketoconazole (or Nizoral), and other prescription drugs. These people may respond more favorably to natural, nondrug treatments.

Side Effects

When the overgrowth of yeast dies, expect discomfort in the first week or so of treatment. Gradually symptoms should decrease and natural treatments can be increased slightly as tolerated. Side effects during treatment may occur due to withdrawal from coffee, alcohol, chocolate, dairy products, sugar, wheat, or the yeast, to name a few. If symptoms go beyond eight days of if they are severe, consult your doctor immediately.

Here is a short list of common problems and methods of partial relief. Rest and relaxation are essential to healing and reduced symptoms.

- Anger and aggression: Take extra vitamin C. Enjoy an Epsom salt bath. Take a walk, exercise, or do deep breathing.
- Cold, coughs, or sore throat: Avoid drafts and damp places. Take vitamin C.
- Cold extremities: Exercise every day; eat warming food.
- Constipation: Eat more vegetables, mainly cooked.
- Depression: Eat properly. Take extra vitamin C, B50-complex, calcium, and magnesium. Vitamins in liquid form are more absorbable. Exercise and reduce your workload.
- Diarrhea: Eat well-cooked whole grains, yams or winter squash, and salads.

- Energy lows: Eat properly. Take vitamin C. Raise body energy levels with exercise.
- Emotional experiences: Eat properly. Take extra vitamin C, B50-complex, calcium, and magnesium.
- Headaches: Take simple aspirin or Advil, if you have to, or feverfew herbs and vitamin C. Avoid cigarette smoke.
- Indigestion: Follow a food-combining diet, and use digestive aids and *L. acidophilus* as needed.
- Mental confusion, spaciness: Eat properly, get enough sleep, and exercise.
- Mucus: Spit it out. The body expels mucus as parasites die.
- Nausea: Avoid citrus and raw salads. Eat yogurt.
- Sleeplessness: Do not eat fruit at night or take vitamin C, *L. acidophilus*, or any strong digestive aid. Avoid chips, meats, or nuts late at night.
- Tooth pain: Take extra vitamin C, calcium, and magnesium
- Excessive weight loss: Be sure to eat two or three meals a day.

Natural ways to speed healing include:

Air purifiers	Laughter and play
Cleanliness, household	Massage
Cleanliness, personal	Meditation
Deep breathing	Positive thinking
Diet and nutrition	Rest
Exercise	Yoga
Fresh air and sunshine	

Ways to support your immune system include:

- Emotional and spiritual: positive attitude, self-love, laughter, affirmations

- Visualization and relaxation: yoga, breathing, meditation, exercise
- Healthful diet: hypoallergenic (rotation if possible), low fat, low sugar, chemical-free, filtered or purified water, adequate digestive function, adequate stomach acid
- Dietary enzymes found in whole foods, vegetables, and fruits
- Antioxidants, vitamins, and minerals found in a healthy, well-balanced diet
- Herbs and other nutrients: garlic, licorice, echinacea, vitamin C, bioflavonoids, vitamin A, beta-carotene, vitamin E, B-complex vitamins, essential fatty acids, and protein

Immune system suppressors include:

- Alcohol
- Allergies
- Chemicals (phenol, formaldehyde, hydrocarbons)
- Air and water pollution; drinking tap water
- Surgery, radiation, and chemotherapy
- Prescription drugs: cortisone, steroids including birth-control pill, NSAIDS (nonsteroidal anti-inflammatory drugs)
- Recreational drugs: marijuana, nicotine, cocaine, amphetamines
- Heavy smoking
- Lack of sleep
- Lack of physical activity
- Airplane travel
- Stress (social, work, financial)
- Depression, bad mood, negative attitude, anger
- Overeating
- High-fat diet
- Excess iron

- Malnutrition (lack of adequate protein; vitamin A; B-complex vitamins, especially B5, folic acid, B6, and B12; vitamins C and E; selenium; zinc; essential fatty acids).
- Nutritional deficiency

Simply follow the dietary changes to enhance your immune system, reducing all known or suspected food allergens, keep stress under control, exercise, practice good hygiene, and get sufficient sleep.

Conclusion
Health Maintenance after Treatment

To prevent a recurrence of *Candida* overgrowth, you must remain vigilant about your diet and lifestyle. The fact that you experienced this illness is a sign that your body, mind, and spirit are more susceptible to *Candida* than others. Recurrence is possible if you let down your guard. Eating the same food day after day is one of the major contributing factors towards food intolerance.

Impaired immunity can result from poor nutrition, but there are other causes like heredity, which plays a major role. Some people seem to inherit an impaired ability to keep infections under control. The treatment followed depends on your body's immune system to finish the job and be healthy.

The usual advice is to support the immune system. Visit your naturopath, holistic medical doctor when you are well, not only when symptoms occur. Health is intimately connected to knowledge; therefore it is important to read about health issues on a regular basis. Millions of people are suffering needlessly, treating chronic illnesses with toxic drugs. The truth is that although we are born with certain genetic tendencies and weaknesses, we do have control over our health and well-being.

What is most important is applied knowledge, which seems to be difficult for most people. People tend to fall into old ways of abusing their bodies. We have to continually eat a healthy diet on a daily basis and remember to keep healthy and strong and not even the overgrowth of yeast will be able to get us down!

Apply the recommendations in this book that you think feel right for you. It is time to substitute many drugs for healthier alternatives. I hope that by having read this book you feel empowered to take control of your health and to use some of the recommendations to heal or control your *Candida* overgrowth forever. Listen to your body and take responsibility for your health. You will feel younger, more fortified, energized, and more in control than you have ever felt in your life.

I wish you all happiness, love, and success.

☆　☆　☆　☆　☆

Focus on health, not disease!

Helpful Resources

United States and Canada

Several resource groups can provide information on various therapies and practitioners. Some can help you find a practitioner in your area.

American Holistic Medical Association
American Holistic Nurses Association
4101 Lake Boone Trail, Suite 201
Raleigh, NC 27607
(800) 878-3373 or (919) 787-5146

American Association of Naturopathic Physicians (AANP)
P.O. Box 20386
Seattle, WA 98102
(800) 235-5800

American Association of Naturopathic Physicians
4435 Wisconsin Avenue, NW
Suite 403

Washington, D.C. 20016
(202) 237-8150
(866) 538-2267 toll-free

Canadian Naturopathic Association
Box 4520, Station C
Calgary, Alberta T2T 5N3
(403) 244-4487

CFIDS Association (for information on chronic fatigue syndrome
and immune dysfunction syndrome)
P.O. Box 220398
Charlotte, NC 28222-0398
(800) 442-3437 or (900) 988-2343 (information line)

The International College of Integrative Medicine
ICIM offers access to its member directory:
http://www.glccm.org/icimed

American Holistic Medical Association (AHMA)
Holistic Medicine
http://www.holisticmedicine.org/

Foundation for the Advancement of Innovative Medicine (FAIM)
www.faim.org

Price-Pottenger Nutritional Foundation
http://www.price-pottenger.org/index.com

National Center for Homeopathy (NCH)
www.homeopathy.org

Michael Biamonte, C.C.N
Certified Clinical Nutritionist (Men)
The Biamonte Center for Clinical Nutrition
(212) 587-2330
info@health-truth.com
www.health-Truth.com

Dan, Natural Health Consultant (Men)
www.yeastinfectionadvisor.com

Rodney Davidson (Men)
www.candida-albicans-cure.com

Master Herbalist
www.blessedherbs.com

Naturopathic Medicine Network
http://www.pandamedicine.com/physicians.html

Dr. Elmer Cranton, MD
Yeast-associated illnesses and treatments
www.drcranton.com

Jack Tips' Do-It-Yourself Lab Tests
Dr. Jack Tips, ND, PhD, CHom, CCN
Natural Medicine
Apple-A-Day Clinic—Telephone consultation for sufferers of *Candida*
www.jacktips.com

Diagnostic labs in the United States and Canada offering a version of fungal antibody tests:

Quest Diagnostics
www.questdiagnostics.com

LabCorp
www.labcorp.com

Genova Diagnostics Laboratory
Candida Immune Complexes and CSDA
(800) 522-4762
www.gdx.net

BioHealth Diagnostics
Blood Test #350—*Candida* DNA and Antibodies
(Chronic *Candida*)

Immunosciences Lab, Inc
Candida albicans Antibodies—Immunity

Diagnos-Techs
Comprehensive Stool and Digestive Analysis—CSDA
(Antibodies, *Candida* antigens in the blood)
(800) 878-3787

Antibody Assay Laboratories
(*Candida antigens* complexes in blood)
(800) 522-2611

Metametrix, Inc
Dysbiosis Metabolic Marker Profile
Organic Acid Test
www.metametrix.com

Medical Diagnostic Laboratories, Inc
DNA/ PCR tests for *Candida albicans*
www.mdlab.com

Meridian Valley Laboratory
Comprehensive Stool and Digestive Analysis: *Candida*
www.meridianvalleylab.com

Vancouver Naturopathic Clinic
www.vancouvernaturopathicclinic.com

Natural Pharmacy and Health Center
www.finlandia.com

Gaia Garden Herbals—Herbal Remedies
2672 West Broadway
Vancouver, British Columbia
(604) 734-4372
www.gaiagarden.com

International Resources

The Great Plains Laboratory
World leader in organic acid testing and evaluating abnormal levels
of yeast
www.greatplainslaboratory.com

Bio-Screen yeast culture test, an urine test for systemic candidiasis
Advanced Nutrition
Broadway House
Tunbridge Wells

Kent, UK TN1 1QU

018 9254 2012

Blood test: A blood test for short-term Candida and long-term Candida:

The Institute of Individual Wellbeing

99 Kings Road

London, UK SW3 4PA

020 7730 7010

fax: 020 7730 7447

Hometest.co.uk

Provides a blood test taken at home and then analyzed for *Candida* and other immune problems

Natural Pharmacy and Health Center

www.finlandiapharmacyonline.com

Books on Nutrition and Vitamins

Prescription for Nutritional Healing

James F. Balch, MD and Phyllis A. Balch, CNC

Avery Publishing Group, ISBN 0895297272

Prescription for Dietary Wellness: Using Foods to Heal

Phyllis A. Balch, CNC

Avery Publishing Group, ISBN 0895298686

Foods That Heal

Bernard Jensen

Avery Publishing Group, ISBN 0895295633

The Candida Albicans Yeast-Free Cookbook
Pat Connolly
McGraw-Hill Companies, ISBN 0658002929

Overcoming Candida: *The Ultimate Cookery Guide*
Xandria Williams
Vega Books, ISBN 1843330423

Candida Directory: The Comprehensive Guidebook to Yeast-Free Living
Helen Gustafson and Maureen O'Shea
Ten Speed Press, ISBN 0890877149

Allergies: Disease in Disguise
Carolee Bateson-Koch DC ND
Alive Books, ISBN 0920470424

Nutritional Supplements and Other Products

Epresat, Salus' liquid multivitamins, including B complex
From health-food stores or order online at www.salus-haus.com

EFA, Essential Fatty Acids in liquid
http://www.bodybuilding.com/store/sun/efa.html

Borage Liquid Gold by Health from the Sun; other products at discount
http://www.vitacost.com

Liquid Health Products
www.mothernature.com

Thorne Research, SF-722
www.thorn.com

Health Products
www.mercola.com

Blood and Skin Rejuvenator, herbal supplement to cleanse and eliminate toxins
www.blessedherbs.com

OmegaZyme, by Garden of Life (digestive enzymes)
www.vitaminsandsuch.net

To Locate a Practitioner:

WESTERN CANADA

Calgary
Dr. Jeoff Drobot, ND
Calgary Centre for Naturopathic Medicine
The Riverside Club
200 - 110 Point McKay Crescent N.W.
Calgary, AB T3B 5B4
T: 403.270.9355
F: 403.237.0747
W: www.calgarynaturopathic.com

Calgary
Dr. Melina Roberts
Advanced Naturopathic Medical Centre
Market Mall Executive Professional Building

Suite 414, 4935 - 40 Ave NW

Calgary, AB, T3A 2N1

T: 403-247-4646

F: 403-247-4660

W: www.advancednaturopathic.com

BRITISH COLUMBIA

Kelowna

Dr. Lorne Swetlikoff, BSc., ND

1451 Columbia Avenue

Castlegar, BC   V1N 1H8

T: 250.365.3326

F: 250.365.3327

W: drswetlikoff.com

Kelowna

Kelowna Naturopathic Clinic

160 - 1855 Kirschner Road

Kelowna, BC V1Y 4N7

T: 250.868.2205

F: 250.868.2099

W: www.natural-medicine.ca

Vancouver

Integrative Healing Arts

Multi-Disciplinary Naturopathic Clinic

730 - 1285 W. Broadway

Vancouver, BC V6H 3X8

T: 604.738.1012

W: www.integrative.ca

EASTERN CANADA

ONTARIO

Mississauga

Dr. Nana Chang, ND

Meridian Naturopathic Clinic & Assessment Centre

2087 Dundas East, Unit# 101

Mississauga, ON L4X 2V7

T: 905.238.9001

F: 905.238.9821

W: www.meridianclinic.com

Mississauga

Dr. Carolyn Kaganovsky, ND

Inner Medicine Naturopathic Clinic

251 Queen Street South

Mississauga, ON L5M 1L7

in the "Village of Streetsville"

T: 905-819-8200

W: www.innermedicine.com

Toronto

Dona-Maria McCowan

Homeopathic doctor

Pacific Health Center

168 Annette Street

T: 416.497.9968

E: dmmccowan@gmail.com

UNITED STATES

ARIZONA

Prescott

Dr. Anthony C. Mulberg, MS, DC, FIAMA

Kachina Healing Center

8363 E Florentine Rd, Suite C,

Prescott Valley, AZ 86314

T: 928.772.4500

F: 928.772.2622

E: drtonym@earthlink.net

W: www.kachinahealingcenter.com

CALIFORNIA

BAY AREA

Berkeley

David Melly, MS, LAc

100 - 2320 Woolsey Street

Berkeley, CA 94705

T: 510.381.4023

E: david@mellyacupuncture.com

W: www.mellyacupuncture.com

Moraga

Farideh F. Naraghi

Quantum Wellness Center, Inc.

55 Carr Drive

Moraga, CA 94556

T: 925.376.2025
F: 925.878.5003
W: ivitalenergy@gmail.com

SAN FRANCISCO

Anatara Medicine
1700 California Street, Suite 520
San Francisco, CA 94109
T : 415-345-0099
E : info@anataramedicine.com
W: www.anataramedicine.com

SOUTHERN CALIFORNIA

San Juan Capistrano
George Weinand
Dorothy Erickson, Naturopath
Neurowaves
27352 Calle Arroyo
San Juan Capistrano, CA 92675
T: 949.363.8250
E: gweinand@neurowaves.com
W: www.neurowaves.com

Laguna Hills
Dr. Ali Meschi, PhD, NHD, CNC
Alternative & Complementary Medicine, Inc.
24953 Paseo de Valencia, Suite 27A
Laguna Hills, CA 92653
T: 949.206.9061
W: www.myholisticdr.com

COLORADO

Boulder
Dr. Kelly Parcell, ND
Dr. Stephen W. Parcell, ND
NatureMed
5330 Manhattan Circle, Suite B
Boulder, CO 80303
T: 303.884.7557
W: www.naturemedclinic.com

WASHINGTON

Renton
Dr. Mark Fredericksen, ND
213 - 2003 SE Maple Valley Hwy
Renton, WA 98057
T: 425.652.2430
E: mark@fredclinic.com
W: www.fredclinic.com

MIDWEST

ARKANSAS

Berryville
Joy Watson
Tom Watson
Osage Natural Health Center
2277 County Road 507
Berryville, AR 72616
T: 870.423.4237
W: www.osagenaturalhealth.com

ILLINOIS

Geneva
Melody Hart, ND, PhD
The Hart Center
127 S. Second Street
Geneva, IL 60134
T: 630.262.5055
W: www.hartcenter.com

Glenview
Dr. Thomas Bayne, DC
Dr. Ingrid Maes, DC
PureBalance
1332 Waukegan Road
Glenview, IL 60025
T: 224.521.1212
W: www.pbhealthcenter.com

INDIANA

Hagerstown
Clean Living Health Clinic
Dr. James Gerni
449 E. Main St.
Hagerstown, IN 47346
E: drgerni@gmail.com
W: www.drgerni.com

OHIO

Salem

Dr. Alan Masters, ND
Nature's Wonders Naturopathic Services
384 Aetna Street
Salem, OH 44460
T: 330.332.1915

MISSOURI

Blue Eye

Joy Watson
Osage Natural Health Center
Blue Eye, Missouri 65611
T : 417-779-0830
W: www.healingtreehealth.net

EAST

NORTH CAROLINA

Dr. Susan Burns

Health and Wellness Initiatives
144 Azalea Circle
Banner Elk, NC 28604
T: 828-221-2324
W: www.healthandwellnessinitiatives.com

NORTHEAST

PENNSYLVANIA

Montgomeryville
Ian Kennedy
Dr. Denise Kelley
True Wellness
577 Bethlehem Pk
Montgomeryville, PA 18936
T: 267.308.0777
E: info@truewellnesspa.com
W: www.truewellnesspa.com

SOUTH

ALABAMA

Madison
Dr. Linda Jarvis, NMD
Jarvis Natural Health Clinic
1489 Slaughter Road
Madison, AL 35758
T: 256.837.3448
E: jarvisclinic@bellsouth.net

FLORIDA

Bradenton
Dr. Gustavo Arrojo, MD
Lifeline Wellness and Longevity Center

2109 59th Street West
Bradenton, FL 34209
T: 941.761.3777

Lake Mary
Dr. Mojka Renaud, LN, Dipl AC NCCA
Holistic Options
101 - 653 Primera Boulevard
Lake Mary, FL 32708
T: 407.333.1059
F: 407.333.4781
E: purehealth@holisticoptionsinc.com
W: www.holisticoptionsinc.com

Palmetto
Dr. John Monhollon, MD
Yvonne Courtney, RN
Natural Health Resource Center
1107 Hwy 301
Palmetto, FL 34221
T: 941.729.1406
F: 941.729.6632

Santa Rosa Beach
Dr. Soto
The Younger You Institute, P.A.
249 Mack Bayou Loop. Suite 201
Santa Rosa Beach, FL 32459
T: 850.267.8452
W: www.yyinstitute.com

Winter Park

Dr. Joya L. Schoen, MD

1850 Lee Road, Suite 240

Winter Park, FL 32789

T: 407.644.2729

F: 407.644.1205

E: jschoenmd@earthlink.net

W: www.midfloridamedicalgroup.com

GEORGIA

Roswell

Dr. Seneca Anderson

Longevity Health Center

2502 Macy Drive

Roswell, GA 30076

T: 770.642.4646

W: www.longevityhealthcenter.com

MISSISSIPPI

Meridian

Thomas Lucky

Meridian's Natural Healing Clinic

1216 Constitution Avenue

Meridian, MS 39301

T: 601.482.2612

TEXAS

Amarillo

ICAM Institute of Amarillo, LLC
1901 Medi Park, Building B, Suite # 1001
Amarillo, TX 79106
T - 806-468-4616
F - 806-468-4618
E: icam@aahsllp.com
W: www.icamamarillo.com

EUROPE

AUSTRIA

Vienna

Dr. med. Walter Glück
Mayrhofgasse 1/24
A-1040 Wien
T: +43-1-5031292
F: +43-1-5031292-20
E: ordination@walterglueck.at
W: www.walterglueck.at

Innsbruck

Dr. med. Andreas Oberhofer
Edith Stein Weg 1
A-6020 Innsbruck
T: +43-512-582964
F: +43-512-579500
E: doc@dr-oberhofer.at
W: www.dr-oberhofer.at

GERMANY

Ahrensburg

Dr. med. Jörn Reckel / Veronika Ehrler

BIMEDICAL

Praxisgemeinschaft für Ganzheitliche Medizin und

Naturheilverfahren

Lohe 1

22926 Ahrensburg

Germany

T: 04102-459945

F: 04102-459911

E: info@bimedical.de

W: www.bimedical.de

Berlin

Medical Center Mommsenstrasse

Mommsenstr. 57

D-10629 Berlin

Province or Country

T : 004930-315173870

E : berlin@kalden.de

Buchloe

Winfried Brinz

Therapie- und Diagnose-Zentrum für Naturheilverfahren

Kloster-Stams-Str. 11

86807 Buchloe

Germany

T: 08241-4153

F: 08241-7858

E: brinzomed@t-online.de

W: www.zentrum-fuer-naturheilverfahren.de

Dortmund

Dr. med Michael Kalden

Praxisklinik für Onkologie und Naturheilverfahren

Westfalendamm 275

44141 Dortmund

Germany

T: 0231-6186741

F: 0231-6186742

E: kalden@kalden.de

W: www.kalden.de

Gägelow

Dipl.- Med. Lutz M. Menzel

Facharzt für Allgemeinmedizin / Chirotherapie

Address Line 2

Marktstraße 1

23968 Gägelow

T : 03841 – 210001

E : info@doc-menzel.de

W: www.doc-menzel.de

Herrsching

Dr. med. Peter Schleuter

Allgemeinmedizin, Homöopathie

Chirotherapie, Osteopathie

82211 Herrsching

Germany

T : 08152-925550

F : 08152-925551

E : mail@arztpraxis-schleuter.de

W: www.arztpraxis-schleuter.de

Ingolstadt

Dr.med. Yasmine Diatzko

Ludwigstr. 1

85049 Ingolstadt

Germany

T : 0841-17881

F : 0841-910118

W: www.diatzko.de

Nottuln

Dr. med. Dipl.-Biochem. Hans-Ulrich Jabs

Facharzt für Innere Medizin

Von der Reck Str. 3

48301 Nottuln

Germany

T: 02502-94080

F: 02502-940821

E: praxis@dr-jabs.de

W: www.dr-jabs.de

Querfurt

Dr. med. Helge Jany, Facharzt für Innere Medizin

Schwerpunkt Gastroenterologie

Homöopathie / F.X.Mayr-Medizin

Nebraer Straße 2 a

06268 Querfurt - Germany

T : 034771/22576

F : 034771/23558

E : info@drjany.de

W: www.drjany.de

SWITZERLAND

Barone Marina & Pascal

Cabinet de Naturopathie

23 Ch. Vi-Longe

1213 Onex - Suisse

T: 022 793.60.77 - 022 793.08.00

C: 079 287.44.35

F: 022 793.08.00

W: www.baronesante.com

Zug

Gesundheitszentrum Vitasol AG Zug

Frau Dr. med. Maricela Fries

Baarerstrasse 18

6300 Zug

Swiss

T : +41 41 729 70 50

F : +41 41 729 70 51

W: www.vitasol.ch

UNITED KINGDOM

ENGLAND

Hant

Dr. Julian Kenyon, MD, MB, ChB

The Dove Clinic for Integrated Medicine

Hockley Mill Stables
Church Lane
Twyford
Hants, SO21 1NT
T: 01962 718000
F: 01962 718011
W: www.doveclinic.com

London
The Dove Clinic for Integrated Medicine
London Clinic
19 Wimpole Street
London, W1G 8GE
T: 020 7580 8886
F: 020 7580 8884
W: www.doveclinic.com

AUSTRALIA

Glen F. Rees BSc, ND
16 Queen St, Warragul, Victoria, Australia 3820
W: www.healthandeternity.com

TURKEY

Dr. Gursel Velioglu & Dr. Banu Ozmen
The LifeCo Well-Being Center
Club Sporium
Cumhuriyet Cad. 4/8
34626 Akatlar
Istanbul, Turkey

T: +90212 325 32 80
W: www.thelifeco.com

SOUTH AMERICA

BRAZIL

Kurotel Longevity Center and Spa
Rua Nações Unidas, 533
Gramado - RS - Brazil
Zip: 95670-000
T: 00 55 54 3295.9393
W: www.kurotel.com.br

http://www.tcolincampbell.org

www.wellnessforum.com

Other resources

Charlotte Gerson
Healing your body the natural way
www.thegersontherapy.com

Dr. Hulda Clark, PhD, ND
The cure of all diseases (including cancer)
www.huldaclark.com

Spring Forest Qigong
7520 Market Place Drive

Eden Prairie, MN 55344

(952) 593-5555

www. springforestqigong.com

Chunyi Lin

Certified in International Qigong (tai chi and Chinese herbal medicine)

Masters degree in human development

Specialities: Holistic health & wellness

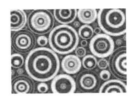

About the Author

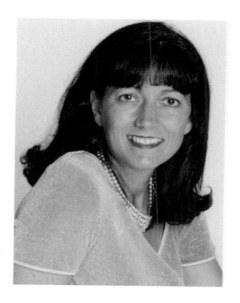

Murielle L. DuBois, ND, RHN

Naturopath and Registered Holistic Nutritionist

Murielle L. DuBois received her Doctor of Naturopathic Medicine Diploma from the Alternative Medicine College of Canada and is also a graduate of the Canadian School of Natural Nutrition. She is a

Registered Holistic Nutritionist and a licensed Cosmetologist with the Cosmetologist Association of British Columbia.

Prior to this, she completed her first year of Bachelor of Arts. at the University of British Columbia. As she was starting her second year, she decided to specialize in alternative medicine, her life-long passion. She did her practicum as a naturopath in holistic health and has been consulting in a range of indications including women's health, digestive concerns, skin problems, *Candida*, fatigue, stress, food allergies, lifestyle guidance, and dietary advice. Through writing, she is dedicated to educating the public because she believes that knowledge is the key component to mindful and healthy living. Her education and clinical experience in preventive medicine enable her to practice medicine that is tailored to the unique needs of the individual.

She believes that personalized preventive care is of utmost importance in helping people achieve their health goals. This includes assisting individuals in regaining and maintaining their health and well-being through natural alternatives and a personalized approach to wellness through a philosophy of simple balance. Physical illness is but an indicator of imbalance on some level of our being and may not be purely physical in origin. Any number of other factors can also influence our physical health, including emotions, lifestyle, environment, and degrees of creativity and personal fulfillment. Health is established when balance is achieved on all levels of our being. Beliefs, attitudes, and motivations can contribute to overall wellness.

The Natural Health Practitioner's Position in Modern and Future Medicine:

The "active sick person" is the first one to bring about his or her recovery or to maintain his or her health. In other words, we must take charge of ourselves with a maximum amount of information.

Natural treatments should be considered as assistance in accelerating the body's own capacity to return to normal. Your body has an incredible ability to heal itself. Sometimes all you need is a helping hand to get things back on track.

None of the recommendations or information contained in this publication should be considered medical advice. The publisher and distributor of this book recommend that you consult a physician before making any dietary change or before implementing new exercise program. While every attempt has been made to verify the information provided in this book, neither the author nor her affiliates or partners assure any responsibility for errors, inaccuracies, or omissions. The responsibilities for any suggestions or procedure described hereafter does not lie with the author, publisher, or distributors of the book.

Further, readers should be aware that the websites listed in this book may have changed or disappeared between when this work was written and when it is read.

Copyright Notice

Information Content Disclaimer

Printed in Great Britain
by Amazon